Exposed

Exposed

The Rise of Extreme Porn and How We Fight Back

Clare McGlynn

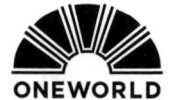

A Oneworld Book

First published by Oneworld Publications Ltd in 2026

Copyright © Clare McGlynn, 2026

The moral right of Clare McGlynn to be identified as the Author of this work has been asserted by her in accordance with the Copyright, Designs, and Patents Act 1988

All rights reserved
Copyright under Berne Convention
A CIP record for this title is available from the British Library

ISBN 978-1-83643-171-8
eISBN 978-1-83643-172-5

Typeset by Geethik Technologies
Printed and bound in Great Britain by Clays Ltd, Elcograf S.p.A.

No part of this publication may be reproduced, stored in a retrieval system, or transmitted, in any form or by any means, electronic, mechanical, photocopying, recording or otherwise, or used in any manner for the purpose of training artificial intelligence technologies or systems, without the prior permission of the publishers.

The authorised representative in the EEA is eucomply OU, Pärnu mnt 139b–14, 11317 Tallinn, Estonia
(email: hello@eucompliancepartner.com / phone: +33757690241)

Oneworld Publications Ltd
10 Bloomsbury Street
London WC1B 3SR
England

Stay up to date with the latest books, special offers, and exclusive content from Oneworld with our newsletter

Sign up on our website
oneworld.co.uk

Contents

	Introduction	1
1	Big Porn	25
2	Harmful Porn	45
3	Rough	69
4	Colour Coded	91
5	Breathless	105
6	Barely Legal	124
7	Family Ties	141
8	Without Consent	162
9	Deepfaked	180
10	Virtual realities	200
11	How We Fight Back	215
	Conclusion: Reclaiming Sexual Freedom and Desire	243
	Acknowledgements	250
	Sources of support	257
	Notes	262
	Index	314

Introduction

'Force' is a searchable category on Pornhub, the world's most popular porn website, visited by 130 million every day. No, it's not, a Pornhub executive told me in 2023. Yes, it is, I replied, as I'd found it the day before and seen titles such as *don't run from me slut* and *she was already shaking but I wasn't done yet.*

That day I also typed 'rape porn' into Google. I was surprised and pleased at what I found. Instead of the pages and pages of rape porn websites that a similar search had brought up a few months before, there were pages and pages of news stories about the harms of rape porn, including links to my research and law reform work. There's a satisfying kind of karma when you realise people search for rape porn and end up with your research talking about how abhorrent it is.

Had Google actually down-ranked rape porn websites, making them harder to find? Perhaps it's just my settings, I thought, and went off to start the same search on another family member's phone, before quickly realising that really wasn't a good idea. The answer is yes, Google has indeed made it more difficult to find rape porn. The websites are still there; they've not been de-indexed (meaning you can't find them at all), just down-ranked so you have to scroll through a few pages to find the material.

This glimmer of hope, however, was quickly squashed when I typed 'force porn'. There it all was, just renamed. Not as obvious as 'rape porn', but it only took a second to think of a synonym for rape – force. To be fair, *'forced'* had been down-ranked, just not 'force'. Though, really, if a company has gone through the effort of down-ranking forced, why not related terms?

Despair set in, but I needed to check out a few more things. I was speaking the next day at a workshop with top 'trust and safety' executives from the largest social media companies and porn platforms. I typed 'deepfake porn' into Google and it returned MrDeepFakes right at the top. This was a notorious website dedicated to creating and sharing AI sexualised deepfakes – where women's ordinary, everyday photos are superimposed into porn without their consent. By 2024, the videos on the site had been viewed over 1.5 billion times.[1] It was getting around 14 million visits a month before it was shut down, largely thanks to Google providing an easy route to weaponise AI tech against women.[2]

My morning on Pornhub and Google was the impetus for this book.

The next day I went to the workshop, where we spent much of the day sharing best practice on preventing or reducing the spread of non-consensual explicit imagery, as well as discussing the need for better education. For me, though, the elephant in the room was the vast empire of pornography, so much of it non-consensual and sexually violent, that was being accessed by millions as we spoke.

It was obvious to me that, while the changes being discussed to reduce the spread of non-consensual intimate images were very welcome, they would ultimately be futile if, at the same time, millions (of mostly men) were choosing to watch non-consensual videos on porn websites and Google was serving up similar material as quickly and happily as a recipe for banana bread. How could we say that we condemned the sharing of sexually explicit deepfakes, when the websites dedicated to creating and sharing them are so easily accessible? How could we be taking rape and other sexual offences seriously when rape porn was being fed to millions as a legitimate genre on the most popular websites? What was the point in expending time and resources on education and training, when as soon as the session ends, the porn websites are there normalising the opposite messages?

Back then, there was very little appetite to talk about the prevalence of porn and the harmful role it is playing in society. My comments landed like a proverbial lead balloon. And I get it. Nobody wants to be labelled a prude or 'sex-negative'; and those promoting, justifying, excusing or ignoring porn seem to have cornered the market as the cool kids in the room. But I felt a certain clarity that day. I knew I needed to try to break the silence, to expose the reality of the porn that millions are consuming. I needed to forge some understanding that to end violence against women and girls, to strive towards equality and liberty for all, to allow everyone to engage in authentic sexual lives, and to improve our democracy and public lives, we must fight back against the pervasiveness and dominance of what I call 'patriarchal porn'.

NOT ALL PORN

The problem is not with porn itself. The problem is patriarchal porn. This is the porn on the largest, mainstream porn websites – often referred to as Big Porn. It's easily discoverable on social media, particularly X/Twitter, and through any search engine. This porn targets heterosexual men and presents a particular way of being a man and having sex that is commonly aggressive, forceful, domineering, degrading and only ever concerned with men's satisfaction. Meanwhile, women are regularly portrayed as unwilling, often humiliated, frequently subjected to violence. When not being coerced, women are shown liking almost anything and everything, no matter how dehumanising. All of this reinforces the social status of women as inferior and existing for the pleasure of men, eroticising gender inequality.

It is patriarchal because these websites are so popular and frequented so often that they are inevitably shaping society's attitudes, culture, laws and policies. It is not niche, or reserved for the dark web, requiring a level of determination to seek it out. It is ubiquitous, and it's sustaining age-old values. By patriarchy, I mean a system structured around men, as a group, whether that be in politics, economics, cultural life or in families.[3] It's a world in which women's interests, rights and dignity are subordinated to those of men. It's a system structured around hierarchies of power, especially those based on race, ethnicity, sexuality and disability. As a result, patriarchy can take many forms, with women from racially minoritised groups experiencing oppression very differently from white women – a dynamic which Audre Lorde calls the 'racist patriarchy'. In eroticising male dominance, it attempts to sell us an unjust system as a desirable natural order. It does this so successfully by transforming gendered inequality into a source of sexual gratification, something attractive and highly enjoyable.[4] Furthermore, eroticising it means that it becomes appealing to both women and men.[5]

Importantly, this is about overarching structures and systems, rather than the choices of individual men (though of course that remains important). Each of us acts within constraints and, as I discuss in the next chapter, Big Porn actively and significantly shapes our actions to suit their business model. It needs to keep us engaged and going back for more, and that means novelty and extremity. The entire success of the porn industry is not because we go back and watch the same video on Pornhub for a few minutes and then return to our working day. It makes billions because it entices us to scroll and scroll, endlessly searching for a new hit, something a bit different. Maybe there's something out there that we prefer? This means prioritising the new, the more extreme, the more divisive content that holds our attention and therefore drives their business. While the PR of Big Porn, and indeed the pervasive message of internet idealism, is about a vast smorgasbord of options for all sexual tastes, satisfying every desire, the reality is an algorithmically driven set of choices designed to hold our attention and keep us coming back.

So this is about societal level change, holding Big Porn to account and demanding change. And the crucial – indeed optimistic – point here is that men's dominance over women is not a natural state of affairs, even if it might seem this way because we are repeatedly told so. Patriarchy is not inevitable. Change is possible.

My focus, therefore, is deliberately on the pornography that dominates mainstream platforms, not on all sexually explicit materials.[6] Pornography is not inherently harmful; people have always created, shared and enjoyed sexual representations. Some refer to 'inegalitarian porn', and those speaking from a public health approach similarly emphasise that 'not all pornography is inherently dangerous'.[7]

Indeed, feminist critiques of pornography have long drawn a distinction between exploitative 'pornography' and 'erotica', understood as sexual expression that foregrounds mutuality, desire and equality. In the 1980s, feminist stalwarts Catharine MacKinnon and Andrea Dworkin defined pornography as sexually explicit material that *subordinates women* – contrasting this with erotica portraying men and women as equals.[8]

Their criticism, therefore, has always been with pornography *as they define it*, not with all sexually explicit content.[9] One of the trailblazers of second-wave feminism in the US, Gloria Steinem, drew a similar distinction, suggesting that, unlike pornography, 'there is likely to be mutual pleasure' in erotica and a 'shared sensuality and a spontaneous sense of two people who are there because they want to be'.[10] Steinem's is just one vision, and any boundaries between erotica and porn will always be porous. But importantly, there are many ways in which sexually explicit imagery can be produced and consumed that do not involve sexual violence, misogyny and racism.

What makes Big Porn so troubling is the particular model it has built: one that rewards violence, misogyny, racial stereotypes and exploitation, because these generate clicks, traffic and profit. This is not an inevitable outcome of sexually explicit expression but the result of a business model that normalises abuse and packages it as entertainment on a mass scale. It stems from a culture that legitimises such practices, facilitating and sustaining them through a lack of regulation.

Therefore, despite the possibility of producing alternatives, what we have seen is the dynamic growth of an industry thriving on shock and aggression. What's lost is the possibility of erotic material that celebrates pleasure without harm. The challenge, then, is not to condemn sexually explicit content altogether, but to demand accountability from the mainstream porn platforms and financial ecosystem supporting them, whose business model depends on misogyny and abuse. What is at stake is not whether people should or should not consume erotica or porn, but whether the dominant platforms should continue to shape our sexual culture through a model that thrives on harm.

Indie and feminist creators have shown that explicit content can be made with care, respect and consent, where performers are fairly compensated, boundaries are honoured and the material is free of harmful practices. If we are to envision a future that values women's sexual freedom and pleasure, it needs to encompass a world where porn can be produced and enjoyed that does not valorise harm – a world of porn without the patriarchy.

FROM EXTREME TO MAINSTREAM

The porn that was once considered extreme is now run of the mill, but we seem not to have noticed, accepting what is out there now as standard, as if it's always been that way.[11] But it hasn't. At the most obvious level, the once controversial nude centrefold in *Playboy* has been replaced by the now easily and freely accessible representations of forced sex available on Pornhub. Decades ago, we used to talk about soft- and hardcore porn, with hardcore defined as including an erect penis. Imagine. That means there was porn without an erect penis. Try finding that today in mainstream porn. Similarly, one of the early studies on the content of porn from the 1990s defined fetish as including 'lingerie' and 'boots'.[12] It's rather quaint.

Incest porn – barely a category two decades ago – is now rife. Similarly, my first research and advocacy work on pornography a couple of decades ago was when we all realised that strangulation porn was easily accessible. The introduction of the *extreme* porn law was designed for that very material. Now, however, we've relabelled it as choking and it's part and parcel of everyday porn. For many younger people, rough porn is not a category, a particular type of porn, it *is* porn. It's just what there is, what is normal. Further, we know that there's far more child sexual abuse material available now than ever before, and that some of this is on mainstream porn websites, sitting alongside the porn imitating child sexual abuse with actors over eighteen but looking very young. Yet few seem to be batting an eyelid.[13]

How did we get here? I've already mentioned the business model, which, in every website and app, prioritises engagement. We know that more extreme content drives greater traffic. This in turn encourages content creators to make riskier content, which is then algorithmically prioritised to secure attention, creating a cycle where ever more challenging content is created and consumed. The algorithmic prioritisation of extreme porn means it's watched more and more, normalising the content and encouraging yet more to be shared. When this content seems standard, we stop noticing what has changed. Imperceptibly, we have become accustomed to what we are seeing, to this ever more boundary-pushing content.

While some try to deflect criticism of porn by denying that we have become desensitised, it is in fact a perfectly normal response to all manner of media and activities. It's got a name: compassion fatigue. With repeated exposure to distressing news, such as reporting of war or famine, we become emotionally exhausted, apathetic or detached. We get used to it and carry on with our lives.

It's also obvious to researchers on pornography, who describe how we all build up a 'tolerance' towards lower levels of aggressive or demeaning sexual acts, requiring more illicit material over time to gain the same sexual stimulation.[14] Indeed, this is what porn users themselves tell us, with one in five in a recent survey acknowledging they are watching increasingly violent and aggressive porn.[15] Members of the public noticed this when taking part in a study with the British Board of Film Classification, which was trying to understand their attitudes towards sexualised violence in films.[16] The participants themselves raised the issue of desensitisation when they realised that this was happening to them and were getting worried about it. I've noticed it myself in writing this book. As well as my conversation with the porn executive about the availability of 'force' porn, I further challenged him about Pornhub having a category *fuck me daddy*. At the time, I was shocked this was so blatantly present, so easily accessible. But honestly, I now see this as rather mild.

Another problem is how this material is presented. Content once explicitly labelled as 'rape porn' has mostly been rebranded. Now it is framed as 'force', or 'accident', involves 'sleep' or 'oops', or includes words like 'don't' in the title. But it's rarely labelled 'rape'. There are no qualms about glorifying sexual activity between parents and their children, though the term 'incest' is seldom used. You can't search for 'child porn', but you can find similar material if you can think of a decent synonym. Such descriptions blur the boundaries of consent, making it more difficult to recognise when abuse or non-consensual acts have taken place.

This relabelling has significant effects as the descriptions and titles of videos play a key role in shaping how we understand the material: what the story is, what message is being sold. Sometimes it's not about what the user actually sees, but how they are encouraged to make sense of it. The titles play a fundamental role in creating the sexual scripts – the key messages – that we take from porn into our daily lives. This is why I share a few of these titles in this book, though most are too shocking and disturbing to reproduce, even though they are the reality of what is being watched by millions everyday. Some of the titles are taken from research I did with colleagues a few years ago into the content on mainstream porn sites.[17] Most though are from 2024 and 2025, when writing this book, and therefore represent up-to-date examples of what is available.

BEYOND 'FANTASY'

Entering this debate can be intimidating. Discussions are often polarised, descending into fruitless barbs about whether or not there is 'direct evidence' that viewing porn leads to committing acts of abuse. Those railing against any regulation of porn claim that there is no scientific 'proof' that porn causes sexual violence, suggesting that should be the end of the debate, since people should get to choose the fantasies they like best. There's no proof that a man watches a violent video and then decides he's going to rape, as we know that sexual offending can't be reduced to a single cause. Few claim that porn directly *causes* sexual violence, and so these arguments are simply knocking down a 'straw man', rather than engaging in the nuanced conversation that is needed.

This is where debates about correlations, risks, probabilities and implications come in. Big Porn has become part of our social world and environment. It plays an active role in shaping sexual attitudes and practices, challenging any idea of media such as porn being pure, private fantasy divorced from any real-world impact. I'm not saying there's a direct, automatic process of viewing porn, and then directly acting it out. But I am saying that rejecting a direct causal relationship is not the same as rejecting *any* relationship. We need to recognise and understand that the media around us, including porn, shapes our choices, decisions and attitudes. Therefore, we can no longer pretend that there are no consequences from millions consuming porn each day. Cumulatively, across society, this porn has become the 'cultural scaffolding' within which each of us make decisions and choices.[18]

Porn therefore is not just a 'fantasy' in someone's head. Firstly, the acts depicted *really* happen, performed by real people, who often suffer as a consequence of their participation in the industry. Moreover, porn seeps into all of our sexual and intimate lives, shaping our preferences and fantasies. It does this through its 'sexual scripts' – the representations, stories and messages that tell us what sex and pleasure are, what is normal, what is to be expected, what we should want, what the boundaries are (if any). Further, the sexual scripts of patriarchal porn create and sustain the underlying conditions within which sexual violence thrives. They normalise acts of sexual violence, making them seem less problematic and, in fact, exciting. They remove an assumption which counters sexual arousal between family members; they push and blur the boundaries of consensual activity between adults and young teenagers.

These blurred lines mean violence against women and girls is not taken seriously in society. Women and girls are left confused and traumatised about what has happened to them, reluctant to tell anyone or report it because they fear (understandably) not being believed. Criminal justice systems struggle to understand the difference between actual non-consent and the eroticisation of non-consent normalised in porn.

The adverse impacts are felt beyond the prevalence and normalisation of sexual violence. Deepfake sexual abuse – where women's ordinary, everyday images are transposed into porn without their consent – is being deployed to push women out of public life. Women's self-censorship in the face of such abuse reduces their visibility in politics and public life, which naturally has an impact on our democracy. In addition, it reinforces the idea that women are there for men's sexual pleasure first and foremost, and that they *ought* to accept anything that a man wants to do to them. This acts to limit women's freedom, constraining their economic futures, and this is all the more profound for Black and racially minoritised women and girls who experience higher levels of online violence and more aggressive forms of deepfake abuse.[19] The flip side is the reinforcement of men's sense of entitlement, superiority, power and control.

If we look ahead, we can see these harms intensifying with generative AI and other emerging tech determining our economic, social and political opportunities as never before, all trained on datasets and an internet awash with misogynistic porn. This plays out through seemingly innocuous phrases such as 'Latina girls' or even 'mummy' being associated with porn and generative AI images reproducing discriminatory norms. What's more, we're seeing the endless drive for more such porn pushing the development of virtual reality and the metaverse – the next, 3D, immersive version of the internet. Misogyny and sexism are not new, but the unbridled rise of AI and virtual reality is catalysing it in novel ways.

FIGHTING BACK

I'm writing this book after twenty years of research, writing and advocacy work on pornography and particularly its legal regulation. As a law professor, my research shines a light on the harmful nature of porn and seeks the best ways to secure justice for victims and hold Big Porn accountable. During the last two decades, I've advised governments, politicians and policymakers on the failings of the law and what we can do about it. I regularly speak in Parliament about my findings, offering actionable recommendations to strengthen regulation. Many of the largest social media companies have sought my advice on how to improve their policies and practices, reducing the harms experienced online by women and girls. I have worked with police to improve their training and guidance, to help them better investigate cases and respond to victims with respect, dignity and care.

Most importantly, I have been honoured to work closely with many survivors of sexual violence and online abuse, understanding their experiences, their ideas of justice, translating their suggestions for change into new law-reform proposals. Similarly, I've learnt so much from the organisations on the front line working to end violence against women, who are so often the first to identify new trends in abuse through their work and who mobilise civil society to insist on reform.

I have advocated for law reforms to tackle all forms of image-based sexual abuse, for better policing, for better internet regulation, for laws constraining extreme pornography. These proposals have had to adapt to the changing political and technological landscape. When I first started working on pornography, the transformative nature of the internet was only just becoming clear. We didn't have smartphones, many of us didn't have computers at home. It's probably difficult to imagine that to get porn you had to go to the corner shop, reach to the top shelf, grab a porn magazine and then confront the shopkeeper with embarrassment. Or you had to go to a grubby side street and enter a sex shop. Perhaps not surprisingly, the drive for more easily accessible porn led to the innovations of the video cassette, then DVDs, then the internet. The rest is history.

I have witnessed first-hand how porn has become so much more accessible, more extreme, and how technology has radically changed our whole world, including our intimate lives. I have seen how fast this can all change, and as I write we are entering the era of generative AI, which porn enthusiasts are already exploiting.

There have been many changes in the course of writing this book. Google finally started to down-rank dedicated 'deepfake porn' websites, although it has been done rather half-heartedly, as we will see. Similarly, it has finally blocked 'force' as well as 'forced' porn, though it took about a year from me first raising it. Maybe in another year we will see more improvements. Just last month, at a meeting with the most senior Google executive responsible for human rights compliance, I pointed out that, while they down-rank 'sleep porn', type in 'asleep porn' and all the same material is there right at your fingertips. It's déjà vu, performative at best.

As a lawyer and academic, I know only too well that law is only part of the solution to all these problems. We need better sex education. We need better porn. We need cultural change. But the law can and does provide the foundations, making clear what is acceptable and what is not. It ensures accountability for platforms and perpetrators; it can give a sense of justice to victims. It can spur change. So while this book may lament most porn, its profound harms and the failures of current law and legal strategies, there is hope.

Imagine a world where the sexual scripts are about women's pleasure as well as men's; where the eroticisation of consent is centre stage; where pigtails, 'tiny teens' and incest are not accepted bases for sexual arousal. Imagine a world where the discomfort of young women in the face of unwanted sexual encounters is acknowledged and legitimised. A world where young teenage boys don't think it's acceptable to 'nudify' ordinary social media images of girls in their class, or their teachers, and then share it among their friends; where their first sexual encounter in the flesh is exciting and satisfying, not a grey version of the porn they are used to. Imagine a world where new tech is not trained on the images, tropes, violence, racism and misogyny of porn, and where liberty-by-design or at least safety-by-design is prioritised from the early stages of technical development.

I want to take steps towards such a world, and the first step involves challenging the idea that mainstream porn is sex-positive for women and girls. Sexual freedom is not secured by chanting the mantra of freedom and handing its interpretation and promotion over to Big Porn. Way back in the early days of *Playboy*, they said ideal women were 'liberated but compliant'.[20] So we had all the rhetoric of freedom, but none of the agency. Fifty years later, little has changed. Dominant ideas of sexual freedom, translated into the language of 'sex-positivity', have reduced the space to challenge the porn industry and prevailing practices.

The pressures and expectations to always be 'sex-positive' about everything and anything have been detrimental to women's and girls' freedoms and opportunities, silencing us when we raise concerns, as few want to be labelled 'sex-negative'. It suppresses inner uncertainty, seeking to persuade young women that feeling disturbed during sexual activity is their problem, not society's, and certainly not porn's. In addition, it inhibits discussions around notions of consent, imposing it as the be-all and end-all of debate, rather than seeing consent as necessary but not sufficient when it comes to what is ethical and welcome in sex.

The rhetoric of sex positivity and porn is exactly that – rhetoric. Anyone suggesting that what you see in Big Porn is about women's sexual pleasure – that it is sexually positive for women – is either delusional or disingenuous. Similarly, in the everyday experiences of women and girls, much sex is consensual but is still experienced as miserable, unpleasant, humiliating, one-sided, painful.[21] This is not about me determining what is right, as if I'm saying only certain types of conventional, old-fashioned sex are good. It's about the women and girls who are sharing their experiences with us, if we listen, including revelations from the studies showing the orgasm gap, with women significantly less likely to climax during a sexual encounter, not just in porn, but in reality.[22] As writer Lucy Morgan has put it in *Glamour* magazine, the 'pervading cultural understanding of pornography is resulting in some of the worst sex we've ever had'.[23] That women are experiencing so much 'misery-making' sex is a profoundly political and social issue.[24] We should be subjecting this sexual environment to scrutiny and asking why we continue to put up with it. It emerges from the gender norms of patriarchy, that men are entitled to sexual gratification at all costs, that women's pleasure does not matter, all embedded in our porn culture.

The pursuit of sexual freedom has to be wrestled away from the stranglehold of Big Porn. Crucially, though, this requires the control and regulation of porn. It won't go away on its own, or without a fight. It needs to be removed from its central role in all of our lives, so that freedom can truly thrive – freedom on our terms, not the algorithmic desire making millions for Big Porn. Regulation, therefore, is essential to liberating women and particularly liberating women's desire.

INTRODUCTION

RECLAIMING SEXUAL FREEDOM

Contrary to common assumptions, it is the liberal values of freedom and liberty, and the protection of human rights, that underpin the necessary regulations. It is not the case that privileging such rights and principles means no regulation of porn. Quite the opposite.

Indeed, my approach begins with nineteenth-century liberal philosopher and proto-feminist John Stuart Mill, whose harm principle underpins many regulatory frameworks in liberal democracies and can justify action here. His idea – that the state should only intervene in an individual's actions to prevent 'harm to others' – is often invoked to argue against restricting pornography. Yet Mill's notion of harm is deliberately broad and can encompass the very real harms produced by today's porn, particularly since his understanding of liberty deliberately centres women's freedom and the need to free them from 'subjection'.[25] Far from opposing regulation, Mill would have been rather keen on controlling the most extreme forms of sexually explicit material.[26]

He insisted that his philosophy was not about the 'unrestricted satisfaction of one's wants and desires', but about the vital precautionary role for law. It's the business of the law to prevent wrongdoing, he said, not to simply to patch up the consequences.[27] This was particularly the case in relation to concerns such as the exploitation of women working in prostitution, which he called a great social 'evil'. He was deeply troubled by the approach of many of his contemporaries, which blamed the women rather than the men who fuelled the demand.[28] He was not convinced by an unbridled freedom to either purchase or sell sex, or state-sanctioned legalisation. Rather, he turned his ire on organised exploitation and those gaining financially from the suffering of others. Therefore, while his thinking was grounded in what were quite radical ideas for his time, his regulatory approach remained liberal, balancing competing interests and safeguarding freedom wherever it was free from coercion or exploitation. His approach – and mine – is captured in his assertion that 'conflicting doctrines, instead of one being true and the other false, share the truth between them'.

A pragmatic, liberal approach, therefore, proceeds on the basis that wholesale bans are rarely appropriate or effective, but that some regulation is vital. This means taking seriously the real harms that flow from porn that reinforces inequality: when women are pressured or coerced, when sexual violence is legitimised and encouraged, when racist stereotypes are repeated, or when sexually explicit deepfakes are used to harass and silence. These are not inevitable features of sexual imagery. They're the result of power imbalances and unjust systems – of patriarchy – which appropriate regulation can address. We need a liberal, pragmatic, political approach that is not grounded in abstract rules but is based on practical goals and in the realities of those experiencing harm.[29]

From this perspective, regulation is not about declaring all pornography oppressive, but about focusing on where it causes most damage – when it erodes women's equal standing in society, restricts their freedom to speak, increases the likelihood of sexual violence and deepens social hierarchies. As US philosopher Martha Nussbaum has explained, it is this type of pornography, rather than sexual expression generally, that directly threatens core ideas of equality and autonomy that are fundamental to liberal societies.[30] A liberal framework can hold two ideas together: that sexual expression can be liberating and joyful, and that it must be limited when it is used to exploit or silence. This balance avoids the extremes of blanket prohibitions on the one hand and total neglect on the other, aiming instead to create conditions where equality, autonomy and justice can coexist.

HUMAN RIGHTS ARE WOMEN'S RIGHTS

One of the main ways these competing interests are navigated is by applying human rights standards. But the dominant focus is very much on defending the rights of (mostly) men wanting to consume porn, with any regulation of tech platforms almost always framed as restrictions on their rights, rather than being essential to securing women's freedom.

We need to reframe these debates. Little is being said about how women's rights are human rights, though some progress is being made. Back in 2015, when I was part of the campaign to criminalise rape porn, Parliament's human rights committee backed us up, agreeing that prohibiting such material 'enhances human rights', rather than restricting them.[31] It wasn't a particularly original idea. We drew on case law from the European Court of Human Rights, as well as United Nations conventions. With Parliament agreeing, and the legislation being adopted, it seemed that a key argument had been won – human rights standards justified the restriction of some forms of pornography. Unfortunately, we've failed to capitalise on this success.

Ten years have passed and we are still having to make the argument that pornography silences women. We must redouble our efforts to explain that when we say 'no', it is often not heard and other times ignored, or misunderstood. Porn and its sex-positivity mantras also stop us from speaking out about disturbing sexual experiences.

Furthermore, its silencing effect goes far beyond our sexual experiences and seeps into our everyday lives, such as the ever-present threat of deepfake sexual abuse. Women's voices are filtered through the norms established by porn: that women are inferior, that their wishes are to be dismissed and ignored, that they are deserving of abuse and humiliation. This is how mainstream porn limits women's speech. Regulation is essential if we do indeed value everyone's right to free expression, not just that of porn-lovers.

The algorithmic power of Big Porn has, in fact, only strengthened free speech arguments in favour of regulation. While there is some talk of regulation as a 'thought-crime', the interactive nature of porn today invalidates any notion of this just being about thoughts without consequences.[32] Even if you 'just' view videos, you are actively shaping sexual scripts by sharing your data, fuelling demand, revealing your preferences. The social role and function of porn, its participatory nature, is undeniable.

Women's privacy rights are threatened by a porn industry thriving on non-consensual porn marketed as a legitimate genre. Once niche, voyeuristic content is normalised online, with a high financial value for 'real' footage. This breaches our privacy rights, encouraging images to be taken up our skirts or down our blouses, making it necessary to check routinely every toilet and every hotel room for hidden cameras.

We need to bring these human rights debates up to date and recognise the central roles of Big Porn and Big Tech in controlling women's speech and rights. This is no longer a private activity, it's a participatory and mainstream one, permeating all aspects of society. It's no longer about prioritising an individual user's rights, but is about recognising the adverse impact on all of us. It's about no longer being duped into believing that Big Porn's freedom ensures our freedom.

THE GOLDEN MEAN

I therefore take a very different stance from religious anti-pornography movements that seek to prohibit all pornography, framing it as immoral, obscene and offensive. There would be no better authority on that than Pope Francis, who talked in 2022 about the 'abnormal consumption of sex on the web' being 'rampant' and an 'attack' on the dignity of men and women.[33] There are also many on the US religious right who talk of banning all pornography to 'restore moral sanity',[34] and these campaigns commonly attempt to control women's reproductive rights and other freedoms. While some of this religious rhetoric co-opts the cause of women's equality, this is a smokescreen for their goal to entrench patriarchal power and control. My focus is on porn as eroticising, glorifying and entrenching gender inequality, not that it might cause 'offence' or is 'immoral' or may encourage people to have sex.

I don't go as far as many feminist colleagues who challenge all forms of pornography as inherently exploitative and underpinning women's oppression. I understand their concerns, and there are many lessons to be learnt from radical feminist thinking on pornography. Indeed, Catharine MacKinnon and Andrea Dworkin were very prescient in calling out the power of the porn industry, talking about how the 'pornographers have convinced many that *their* freedom is *everyone's* freedom'. This is exactly what Big Porn has successfully done. Nonetheless, I want to hold space for sexual representations that are liberating, and for pursuing a more pragmatic agenda for change.

So my approach seeks the 'golden mean', some balance between polarised positions. It's a difficult place to be. Back in 2007, the first seminar I organised with colleagues on the extreme pornography law brought together radical feminists, Feminists Against Censorship, organisations representing the BDSM community, free speech scholars and many more from across the political spectrum. Bringing together this diversity of views was thought so unusual that *The Times* sent journalist Andrew Norfolk (who would later expose the Rotherham sexual exploitation grooming gangs) to report on it, describing us as a group from 'law professors to bondage aficionados'.[35] We'd simply wanted to foster debate and seek some common ground.

But occupying the middle ground is a real challenge. Big Porn, male influencers and dominant liberal thinking frame these issues as binary – sex negative/positive, free speech/censorship – silencing critics as prudish or fuelling a 'moral panic'. Arguments differentiating between particular forms of porn and laws are usually (deliberately) ignored. The label 'pro-porn' also masks nuance, as some producers, performers and writers are similarly critical of Big Porn and so are not pro any and all porn, but only indie, ethical, feminist porn.[36]

LIBERATING DESIRE

All this is to say that the liberal values of freedom and liberty, and the rights of free speech and privacy, justify regulating patriarchal porn. This is in the negative sense of freedom from harm, as well as the positive sense of freedom to flourish, liberating our desires. In fact, the pro-porn and do-nothing lobbies are reactionary and regressive, seeking to preserve the rights of multi-million-dollar platforms to shape our behaviour in ways that are seriously harmful.

After all, the porn we are being fed is deeply illiberal. There is nothing progressive about championing porn where racism is rife and blatant. There's nothing progressive about porn where women's pleasure is ignored; where women are coerced; where sexually violent porn is commonplace; where we are encouraged to gain sexual gratification from visualising sex with very young-looking girls. There's nothing progressive and liberal about a regulatory regime that enables search engines, social media platforms and payment providers to facilitate this misogynistic porn, serving up rape and incest porn as readily as puppy videos. Effective regulation is therefore not about policing sexual expression, but about dismantling an industry that weaponises pornography to suppress women's liberty and freedom.

Therefore, while those who celebrate this porn and reject regulation claim to be the protectors of liberal values, they are not, and they are certainly not defenders of women's autonomy and liberty. This book challenges the liberal defence of pornography on its own terms, arguing that it is essential that we regulate it and by doing so transform the pornography landscape. Reclaiming these liberal values are essential to reclaiming our sexual lives, our sexual freedom and securing greater equality and liberty for us all.

I

Big Porn

WE'RE WATCHING IT ON THE BUS, THE TUBE, ON THE PLANE instead of the inflight entertainment. We're watching it in libraries. We're watching it at the office, or at home when we're supposed to be working. We're watching it at school. We're even watching it in Parliament.

Big Porn is the master manipulator, infiltrating and scripting our lives to such an extent that it's almost unnoticed. It's the cultural and political wallpaper surrounding us. Even if you think you're immune – 'I don't watch it', you might say – you're not. Rest assured that every day you are almost certainly mixing with people who do, whether that be your children and family members, work colleagues, fellow commuters, friends and acquaintances. And beyond those you mix with, Big Porn is embedded in the lives of those who make decisions that affect all of our daily lives, the politicians, businesspeople, executives running internet platforms, content moderators, criminal justice personnel, the media.

You may think I'm exaggerating. Let me try to show that I'm not. Let's start with some statistics. Globally, each day, Pornhub gets around 130 million visits.[1] And it's not just Pornhub. In 2022,

XVideos attracted 3.32 billion visits per month and XNXX, 2.5 billion.² Across the European Union, these three largest porn platforms, together with Stripchat, have over 45 million average monthly users.³ Another way to think about this is by comparisons with some household names. The top three pornography websites are visited more often than the likes of Amazon and Netflix.⁴

Thinking about the UK particularly, one third of adults visit porn websites each month.⁵ They're mostly men (73 percent), equating to 10.1 million men. Pornhub is by far the most popular site, meaning that, throughout 2023, one in four adult men in the UK visited it.⁶ Another way to understand the cultural significance of Pornhub is to realise that, in December 2024, just one month, there were 185 million visits to Pornhub from the UK.⁷

Access to these sites is mostly via smartphones; it's obvious really, but it's the ease of access that explains both the increase and the normalisation.⁸ You can access it on your phone, in the same way you switch between emails, social media and music – mindless scrolling when we are bored or in want of distraction. It's no longer a private, discreet activity. It's mostly free, with only a very small proportion requiring payment.

WHO IS RESPONSIBLE FOR BIG PORN?

The companies with a strangle-hold on the market are Pornhub, owned by Aylo, a Canadian multinational porn company that also owns many other porn sites including Redtube, YouPorn and Brazzers. There are other popular platforms, such as XVideos, XNXX and XHamster, which similarly dominate the rankings of most popular websites. Google plays its part in sustaining the world of porn by facilitating easy access to a range of sites, such as those featuring incest or rape porn. It serves up porn whenever it can, knowing this drives engagement.

Then there are some of the largest social media sites, the most important being X, which is awash with pornography. There are platforms hosting pornography whose terms of service prohibit it, such as Reddit, Twitch and Snapchat. Newly emerging social media sites such as Bluesky allow porn, but at the moment you have to wade through so many satirical comments about porn before you actually get to the real stuff that I suspect anyone genuinely searching for porn will be quickly put off (for now).

These social media sites play a significant role in sustaining the porn industry. For many teenagers, X provides their first foray into porn.[9] Teenage boys particularly are using X, with the express intention of sourcing videos directly from porn actors, which they think is more 'realistic' than content on adult sites.[10] Even on sites ostensibly banning pornography, such as Instagram, it is still pushed to young boys, including invitations and direct links to paid-for adult sites and services.[11]

The material on X is often more extreme than that on Big Porn, and because it is on a social media site, it is seen as lawful – it's on X, so it must be OK. Their terms of service say that users must not upload 'content promoting exploitation, nonconsent, objectification, sexualization or harm to minors, and obscene behaviours'. But there's a clear mismatch between what is supposedly prohibited and what is allowed on the site.

I'm not, in this book, focused on smaller platforms producing indie, ethical or feminist porn, though I discuss these genres later.[12] I'm not focused on queer porn, which rarely features on mainstream platforms and raises very different issues around users, impacts and empowerment.[13] While there is some gay porn on the mainstream sites, that material requires specific analysis and is a small part of the sites overall. And the lesbian porn available on these sites is hardly ever about the sexual pleasure of women, instead catering to men's fantasies of lesbianism.

The dark web is beyond my scope. Sure, there is some truly awful stuff there, but regulating that is another issue. I'm also not specifically addressing child sexual abuse material, as this category is already illegal, though this is part of the discussion about incest and teen porn. My focus is on the English-language porn sites available predominantly across Western societies. If accessing porn from parts of the Middle East, India and Africa, debates are different in terms of accessibility, and the nature of the content, particularly around racism, ethnic tensions and misogyny.

What about OnlyFans and similar sites? OnlyFans exploded into the public consciousness during the pandemic. It's primarily a platform for sex workers, though the company loves to tell us that there are lots of recipes and pictures of pets. The key difference with OnlyFans is that it operates behind a paywall. You have to seek it out, pay for it and thereby disclose (some of) your identity.

After many concerns over access and content, OnlyFans has gone on a trust and safety offensive, introducing policies around the consent of everyone in videos, and tightening access requirements such as proof of identity. Nonetheless, serious questions remain about its moderation policies and the material available.[14] Does it host some of the same sort of vile content that I will be discussing? Almost certainly. I'm not giving it a free pass. It is a huge corporation exerting influence on our political and cultural world and not in beneficial ways. Its very existence tells us a lot about our society. But it does provide greater agency and control for those working on the platform, and it is behind a pay wall, meaning that it is not freely and easily accessible to everyone. For this reason, few of us know what's on there. There is a need for further investigation into its content, but for now, my focus is on the free-to-access mainstream sites.

THE CHILDREN OF PORNHUB

A challenge to mainstream porn was made in December 2020, when the *New York Times* published an article titled 'The Children of Pornhub' by the award-winning journalist Nicholas Kristof.[15] He highlighted how videos of rape, voyeurism, child abuse and other forms of assault had been uploaded to Pornhub without consent and downloaded millions of times. Kristof drew on the tireless work of campaigning organisations like the UK-based #NotYourPorn, survivors who courageously shared their stories and international movements targeting Pornhub, including Laila Mickelwait's #TraffickingHub.[16] The article lit a flame worldwide, drawing attention to Pornhub's role in profiting from illegal and exploitative content. Very quickly, Pornhub realised it had to make significant changes and removed about ten million videos.

One year later, Kristof targeted XVideos with a similarly evocative *New York Times* piece entitled 'Why Do We Let Corporations Profit from Rape Videos?'[17] XVideos were continuing to profit from hosting child sexual abuse material and rape videos and were doing little about it. He bolstered his argument by referring to my research with colleagues into the content on mainstream porn websites.[18] We had found that one in eight titles on the front pages of the most popular porn websites described sexual violence, and this included XVideos.

Survivor testimonies were at the heart of the article. Kristof shared the story of a young Australian woman who took her own life after the unbearable humiliation and abuse she'd experienced when a nude she'd shared with a trusted boyfriend ended up on XVideos and other porn sites around the world, and she found great difficulty getting it removed. These are the stakes, Kristof said, posing the question: do we side with her, or with XVideos?

Since these articles and worldwide outcry, Pornhub has been on a PR offensive. It renamed its parent company but while the ownership officially changed, the management remained much the same. Two executives moved on; the rest are still there. Pornhub claims that trust and safety is at the heart of all they do.[19] Indeed, I've heard the full spiel myself from the lead for trust and safety and the head of brand and community appointed to restore the company's reputation. And things have changed, to some extent. There is improved verification of uploaders, some of the most extreme searches are blocked and they work closely with trusted flaggers like the UK's Revenge Porn Helpline to remove non-consensual material. But the content on their sites continues to include illegal material and promote non-consensual acts, and incest videos are rife.

Pornhub was forced to act by Mastercard and Visa. The credit card companies themselves faced public scrutiny after the *New York Times* articles due to their role in facilitating the illegal activities and, indeed, the fact that they too had known what was going on and had, until the publicity, failed to act. They finally withdrew their payment processing, effectively cutting off a significant portion of Pornhub's revenue stream and initiating the changes at Pornhub. Similarly, it was only when Kristof named PayPal as still providing payment services for XVideos that PayPal removed their services from that site.

But what now? Multiple lawsuits continue against Pornhub, and against the payment providers, for facilitating the ongoing abuse of so many women and girls by repeatedly refusing to take down the illegal videos.[20] Some cases have been settled, but Pornhub continues to fight many more. Not only are they defending the cases brought by abuse victims, but they commonly challenge any regulation that might reduce their profits.[21] They are challenging the attempts by the European Union to implement a new legal regime regulating the very largest online platforms. It would be comical if it weren't so serious: Pornhub, together with porn sites Stripchat and XVideos, is trying to claim that they don't pass the regulatory threshold of 45 million monthly users across the whole European Union.[22] You can bet that's not what they're telling their advertisers. The European Commission was unimpressed and, in May 2025, opened a formal investigation into Pornhub and other platforms for breaches of their obligations under the Digital Services Act.

Don't be fooled by a very effective PR machine suggesting change at the heart of Pornhub's parent company, Aylo. Big Porn has been dragged kicking and screaming into some minimal efforts at legal compliance. But its patriarchal core remains the same.

BIG TECH AND OUR ALGORITHMICALLY CURATED LIVES

Big Porn is one head of the hydra Big Tech. Big Tech profits from the attention economy – the time our eyes are glued to the screen. We know this from Big Tech's own documents. Frances

Haugen blew the whistle on Facebook in 2021 when she released internal documents affirming that their algorithm feeds users 'more and more divisive content in an effort to gain user attention and increase time on the platform'. It could not be more plain. One confidential Facebook presentation stated: 'Our algorithms exploit the human brain's attraction to divisiveness'.[23] Big Tech feeds us – there's a reason it's called our 'feed' – information designed to elicit an emotional response from us, because that's what keeps us engaged. Negative emotions such as fear and anger are more easily prompted, and dwell in us longer than positive ones, so engagement is naturally premised on encouraging and sustaining these negative emotions and impacts. Plus, people on the extremes are more predictable in what they like and want, and algorithms thrive off predictability. Pushing us to extremes makes both technical and financial sense, with companies generating profit through advertising and data mining. This is algorithmic content maximisation, filtering, ranking, categorising, all driven by the need to maximise the profit that comes from maximising our time on the platforms.

What's the impact of this business model? As one former Google executive aptly writes, technology is hijacking our minds.[24] Companies pay vast sums to Big Tech to buy the data in order to learn from and thereby control our tastes and behaviour. As well as being part of the attention economy, these firms are part of 'surveillance capitalism' – generating profits through capturing and selling our personal data and every aspect of our preferences.[25] Vast sums are then spent on targeted advertising because it influences us; we change our behaviour as a result. As tech guru and former Microsoft executive Jaron Lanier makes clear: 'it is the gradual, slight, imperceptible change in your own behaviour and perception that is the product. That's the only thing there is for them to make money from. Changing what you do, how you think, who you are.'[26] Lanier calls Big Tech 'behaviour modification empires'.[27]

They know this. This is the whole raison d'être of these platforms. Back in 2017, the first president of Facebook, Sean Parker, talked about how the content on social media 'literally changes your relationship with society, with each other', and then said, 'god only knows what it's doing to our children's brains'.[28] Facebook knows precisely how harmful it is to the well-being of so many, including teenage girls. One of the released Facebook internal memos starkly revealed its complicity in the growth of eating disorders: 'We make body image issues worse for one in three teen girls'.[29] Despite the headlines, little has changed in concrete terms. If anything, we are getting less and less bothered by it. In late 2024, yet another study found that Instagram (owned by Meta/Facebook) still fails to remove self-harm content for teenagers, and its algorithm was still actively contributing to the formation and spread of self-harm networks.[30] Sadly, this report received hardly any public attention.

We can see that social media content *shapes* our interests much more than it reflects them. As writer Adele Zeynep Walton writes, algorithms are today's culture makers, norm providers and thought-leaders.[31] These are vast, algorithm driven, user-generated platforms changing our behaviour, and this is deliberate. After all, that's how Big Tech makes money. Now, after decades of research into algorithmic harm, there's a growing consensus that we need to regulate Big Tech. Across the global north, we've seen the adoption of legislation such as the UK's Online Safety Act (2023), the EU's Digital Services Act (2022) and Australia's

Online Safety Act (2021). These regulations all impose obligations on the largest websites regarding the content they host.

WHAT DOES THIS MEAN FOR PATRIARCHAL PORN?

It isn't a stretch to see that everything we say about Big Tech applies to Big Porn.[32] The porn industry looks more like Silicon Valley than the Playboy Mansion, full of tech bros with expertise in algorithms, advertising, data mining and search engine optimisation.[33] These are not creative filmmakers trying to reimagine who and what porn is for. Porn is simply the way to make billions.

But the situation is far worse than in relation to Big Tech, where the business model is clear. With porn, the internet idealism remains strong: the anticipation that the internet would open up new genres of porn to many more people, facilitate indie and feminist porn, democratise porn in a way that might maximise sexual freedom, particularly for those with diverse sexualities. Instead, internet porn quickly became a serious business enterprise when the original owners of Pornhub saw the opportunity to create the YouTube of porn, a website where anyone could upload anything and have it all in one place. Again, this might sound great. But while individuals were celebrating this opportunity to share their porn with the world, and others relished seemingly being able to watch any porn they wanted, the porn-trepreneurs have different priorities.

The free porn websites began to drown out the activity of independent, ethical porn creators. In fact it was their material that was now getting uploaded to the free porn sites, without their agreement, and contrary to copyright laws, but what could they do?

As soon as they complained, someone else was uploading it again. Soon, these sites became the only place to showcase your work, alongside the amateur porn and alongside the child sexual abuse material, the rape videos and other non-consensual pornography. Pornhub monopolised this new way of distributing and making money from porn, changing the industry forever.

Big Porn, like social media platforms, is tracking and monitoring our visits, profiling us so as to keep us coming back. This includes placing a monetary value on every video tag. Documents released as part of the litigation against Pornhub reveal that the company kept financial data on tags such as 'teen', one of the most profitable categories, as well as on 'extra small petite teen' and 'very very young girl'.[34] (Tags are the labels used to describe a video, and are given either by the uploader, or the website, or both, and then used to facilitate searches via an algorithm.)

Adverts are obviously crucial, with estimates of 4.6 billion daily ad impressions on Pornhub earning the company hundreds of millions of dollars.[35] These are not adverts for breakfast cereal, cars or some other anodyne product. Many are for other forms of porn that are themselves concerning, such as adverts for a 'family sex-simulator porn game' promoting sexual activity with other family members.[36] Another ad tells users that 'in these games you will fuck more bitches than you ever saw in porn'.[37] Further, despite claims that they don't allow image-based abuse material, adverts for nudify apps – to produce nudes from clothed images of women without consent – continue to be promoted on mainstream porn sites and social media platforms.[38]

The content available is extreme, divisive and boundary-pushing by design. We get hooked on the extremes of sexuality precisely because they are unusual, and spark unease and discomfort in us.

And the algorithm prioritises the content people keep coming back to, meaning the extreme users play a part in determining what is presented to the rest of us. This is not reflecting an authentic idea of what we are interested in, nor is it an accurate representation of the full range of human sexuality.

This type of content is needed because Big Porn has to have something to market, advertise and push, and viewing two (or more) people having joyous sex is not enough, not sufficiently different, marketable, categorisable. It has to be boundary-breaking, challenging, body-punishing and taboo-busting, and it has to play into ancient tropes and stereotypes. This also happens through the labelling process, with shock-value tags and recommendations receiving more attention, therefore keeping you engaged longer. Sites insist on these tags, and offer related and more salacious tags when uploading; they know what their users click on, and so the vicious cycle continues.

Porn sites draw you in with landing pages overloaded with images, titles, options, adverts and gifs. Researchers call this 'panicked arousal', making you feel like you to have to keep clicking, looking, searching.[39] It's all very deliberate. The design draws your eye clockwise, a cyclical viewing pattern that compels you to browse the entire space, to check out all the options, as part of the standard design for marketing.[40] You hover over an image and it plays, with a whole new set of adverts and options, making you feel in control, giving the illusion of choice, though it is all algorithmically generated.

It's mesmerising. You become tantalised by the prospect of the perfect image or video, though this is imaginary, rendering every image inadequate. But what we forget, or do not realise, is that this is all pre-determined. We forget what we initially wanted.

Zahra Stardust writes about how algorithmic tagging and ranking systems in Big Porn benefit white performers and rank far lower Black, brown and Indigenous performers.[41] Another study examined thousands of videos and home pages presented to new users to show how the Pornhub algorithm uses rigid categories of gender, sexuality and interests, contrary to the assumption of almost infinite variety and tastes.[42] Nuance costs money.

And it is equally important to realise that this is a two-way process. Another way in which Big Porn has transformed the industry is through participation and community forums. This is 'participatory porn', where every view fuels the algorithms and shapes the content, and where the platforms encourage membership, allowing users to interact with each other and the content through likes, comments and tags. Some even include engagement with the porn actors. This is where we see the inter-relationship with social media platforms, with thousands sharing online their favourite videos from the porn sites.

Mutual reinforcement has become vital to the process. There is no situation where an individual user watches a video and then wonders what others think, whether they are the only one watching it, questioning whether they should be doing this. All the information in front of them tells them they are not alone, that they are right to enjoy it, and they can easily find online groups and forums to further indulge their particular predilections. They might not participate further, but in the mere watching, they have contributed to the community understanding and meaning, and what is then in turn reproduced by content creators and the algorithms. Participatory porn: not just private thoughts or fantasies, but engagement and active reinforcement.

Therefore, just as we accept that Big Tech is changing our behaviour – more political polarisation, more eating disorders, more harassment – Big Porn is doing the same, threatening our sexual freedom. If it wasn't changing our behaviour, Big Porn simply would not be making so much money. Thus, the profound paradox is that, while online pornography is championed as expanding our sexual autonomy, it in fact diminishes it. It shapes our desires in ways that meet commercial needs and encourage more extreme and contentious content. Sexual content is categorised, tagged and labelled within the parameters of what sells and how fast. The reality therefore is that the shift of pornography to algorithm-driven porn platforms, most of which are controlled by one company, poses a threat to our individual autonomy and our sexual culture.[43] This is not just Big Tech selling us more stuff we don't need; it's *constructing* our sexual desires to keep us coming back and searching for more. We are being duped by Big Porn to think, feel and act in certain ways.

THE BIG PORN AND BIG TECH COLLUSION – 'IT STAINS YOUR BRAIN'

Big Porn and Big Tech are not two parallel internets. They collude in encouraging and sustaining a patriarchal world. Flip between Pornhub and internet memes on your social media and all is well; what you see in porn is not actually uncomfortable and disturbing, as it's being normalised across YouTube, TikTok and other social media. Certainly, that is the case if you are a young man or boy.

We know at this point that the 'manosphere' is a vast network of men's communities promoting specific forms of hyper-masculinity, misogyny, sexist beliefs and opposition to anything vaguely feminist.[44] This is AI-manipulated masculinity – AI influencers,

AI girlfriends, AI sexual therapists, AI pimping, all algorithms pushing oppressive content. These groups can be found on popular social media platforms such as YouTube, with its 'watch next' algorithm recommending increasingly sexist content to keep users engaged.[45] They thrive on Reddit and TikTok, where influencers – sometimes now called 'manfluencers' – shape debates and ideas.[46]

The men in the 'manosphere' tend to blame women and feminists for most of society's problems. When investigators set up a fake account on TikTok of a thirteen-year-old boy, they were quickly directed to content from one of the most notorious manfluencers, Andrew Tate. In one video, Tate described how he expects his girlfriends to behave: 'I inflict, I expect, absolute loyalty from my woman,' he says. 'I ain't having my chicks talking to other dudes, liking other dudes. My chicks don't go to the club without me, they are at home.'[47] Plus, he's on record celebrating choking/strangulation during sex, and has been accused of rape and trafficking, illustrating the correlations between harmful porn, organised crime and the manosphere.[48]

This is not about a small and marginal group of men with little impact on the rest of us. The manosphere *is* social media for so many, particularly younger men and teenagers. You can't escape it, even if you wanted to. So, while we talk about the manosphere and manfluencers, it might be better just to talk about online content being fed to and consumed by men, and young men in particular.

Researchers who set up new accounts on YouTube, with no hint of interests or preferences, were almost immediately recommended anti-women content, including various high-profile influencer 'take-downs' of 'feminist arguments'.[49] Much of the anti-women material was not explicitly labelled as such, instead having names like 'money tips' and 'learning attitude'. By day four, these new accounts were being recommended neo-Nazi material and content mocking LGBTQ+ activists. This content is actively promoted to millions, without any opposing perspectives, and it only gets more extreme.[50]

TikTok is much the same.[51] When opening accounts identifying the owners as young men interested in sports and video games, they were fed misogynistic content in less than fifteen minutes. After two to three hours, it was dominating the feed, together with conspiracy theories and spurious advice on mental health and wealth accumulation. Most recently, a BBC investigation showed how a sixteen-year-old boy was served violent and misogynistic content including videos of someone being hit by a car, a monologue from an influencer sharing misogynistic views, and clips of violent fights. He tried to use the tools on Instagram and TikTok to say he was not interested in this content, but it kept coming. He talked about another video making light of domestic violence, an image of a woman with bruises and the caption 'My Love Language'. He said all this horrific content 'stains your brain'.[52] You can't stop thinking about the images, he said, and then they seep into everyday life, with friends talking about what they see online, trying to make sense of it.

There is a growing gap between young men and women's political orientations, with many men veering towards more extreme, right-wing politics dominated by authoritarian, patriarchal leaders.[53] This is a worrying change, given that younger people used to be more progressive, particularly in relation to gender equality and women's rights.[54]

For people like me, who for decades have worked in service of gender equality, our faith has always been placed in the younger generation. We thought, in time, things would improve. But we're now seeing the reverse. Young men report feeling it's harder to be a man than a woman.[55] But young women feel the exact opposite. As I write this chapter, a new report has been published warning of the rise of misogynistic culture spread by influencers such as Tate, with the UK government's anti-extremism tsar warning of the 'growing normalisation of harmful attitudes toward women among young men, particularly within schools'.[56]

These emerging differences in political allegiances became even more stark during 2024, with younger men being far more likely than young women to vote for Donald Trump.[57] In the US election in particular, the influence of the right-wing manfluencers was clear.[58] This follows a shift in voter patterns across Europe, with younger men similarly moving towards more extreme and right-wing politicians.[59] In the UK, younger men were far more likely than young women to vote Conservative or Reform.[60]

Young men are understandably concerned about their lives, their prospects and the state of the world around them. Their understanding of their role in society, and of what it is to be a man, is unstable. There's heightened polarisation based on race, with young Black men being targeted and scapegoated in a society barely able to conceal its prejudice. Young working-class men feel a sense of betrayal, still living under the long shadow of deindustrialisation. In many of the UK's regions, skilled jobs have not replaced those once offered by Britain's factories, and young men feel trapped in an economy built on insecure, low-wage work. The manosphere and its influencers appeal because they speak to the realities faced by young men – alienation, economic failure, loneliness and a dim vision of the future. In these conditions, many men are angry and resentful that the prospects promised to them by society and experienced by the older generations – social mobility, economic and social influence – have not materialised and in fact may be going backwards.

There is no issue with raising these concerns. The problem lies in its diagnosis of the causes, with the manosphere's fixation on women and girls, on their caricature of feminism, of their zero-sum claim that suggests women's empowerment must necessarily equate to men's disempowerment, supposedly evidenced through pseudo-scientific theories about men and women's natural preferences and qualities.[61]

The manosphere channels men's anger not to the authoritarian, capitalist political systems that have promoted economic polarisation, racism and individualism – but at women. They are being fed a narrative that does not blame the politics and economic policies that have led us here, but instead blames feminism.

What we are seeing is mutual reinforcement between the manosphere and patriarchal porn, promoted and facilitated by Big Tech. This porn privileges men's sexual entitlement over women's, privileges heterosexuality, presents force and coercion as normal (and idealised) characteristics of masculinity and renders anyone who is not white as other, to be fetishised. Simultaneously, the manosphere reinforces these ideas about men's role and entitlement. It sometimes does this explicitly, talking about how women should be treated, and about sex as punitive, with women compliant.

This means that young men can watch influencers valorising choking or strangulation on social media and then switch apps to see this promoted in porn. It's seamless, interconnected. Indeed, a study of the chat rooms in some of the more extreme misogynistic online communities compared them with mainstream porn and found distinctly worrying similarities and overlaps in language and attitudes.[62]

Overall, this leaves us with the paradox that, while institutional, structural power continues for men as a group, many individual men feel powerless. The union of men's interests and capitalism via Big Porn and Big Tech offers men ways to feel less threatened and more powerful.[63] Choking/strangling a sexual partner, literally having their well-being, possibly their life, in your hands, is a power trip. Feeling financially insecure? Why not watch exploitation porn where women with no money agree to have sex with you? Concerned about women's supposed advancement at your expense? Feel better by watching porn with men spitting on them, gagging them, calling them bitches and having sex when they are drugged or asleep. I'm not saying these are conscious choices (though some might be). But this is the dark underbelly, the reality of what it means when Big Tech and Big Porn are two sides of one coin, mutually reinforcing each other, all in the name of making more and more money.

THE MASTER MANIPULATOR

The great PR success of Big Porn is that visitors to these sites feel completely in control of their viewing experience. We think we are choosing what to view, what to click on next, but everything is by design. The imperceptible shifts, nudges, offerings mean we don't notice where we go. This is recognised in research into the pathways from child sexual abuse material to contact offending, noting that there's rarely a psychological threshold to cross or moral challenge to consider.[64] There's no sudden leap from the acceptable to the deviant. This is the same for more and more extreme manosphere content and mainstream porn.

Big Porn is the master manipulator. We are the frogs, slowly being boiled alive.

While we are better informed about the trappings of Big Tech, Big Porn is lagging behind. We either don't notice or we turn a blind eye. We don't go there, don't want to be seen to (supposedly) trample on people's private lives, even though it is the porn companies that are harvesting and selling our data. We don't want to be labelled censorious or prudish or whatever other negative label is commonly attached to those who challenge the porn industry. We're too embarrassed to talk about sex. We don't want to accept that what we are being fed is not our choice, that our desires are shaped by algorithms sending us down rabbit holes into more harmful content. We don't want to face these realities. But we must.

2

Harmful Porn

SINGER BILLIE EILISH MADE HEADLINES A FEW YEARS AGO WHEN she talked about her experiences of growing up watching porn. 'I think it really destroyed my brain,' she explained. 'I feel incredibly devastated that I was exposed to so much porn … it led to problems where, you know, the first few times I had sex I was not saying no to things that were not good. And it's because I thought that that's what I was supposed to be attracted to.'[1] Like every other young person, she'd thought pornography was 'how you learned how to have sex'. The 'real problem,' she said, is that porn skews wider understandings of what's normal during sex.

Typically, the outcry was not so much about porn having such a devastating impact on many young people and so perhaps we should do something about it. Rather, it was Eilish challenging the dominant view that porn is a liberating, 'sex-positive' fantasy. Eilish herself said she'd originally felt 'really cool for not having a problem with pornography'. Disputing porn's positive impacts resulted in Eilish facing criticism and abuse, not only from the porn industry but from the broader establishment view that porn is an untouchable right and good.

Nonetheless, young people are beginning to find the strength to speak out. In a recent study by the Children's Commissioner, one young woman expressed her dismay at the impact of porn on young boys, saying: 'it alters their reality'.[2] When I first read this, I was struck by this insight. Young men too are beginning to wonder about the role of porn, with one 21-year-old explaining, 'it can lead you down dark paths'.[3]

Similarly, we see women in their twenties and thirties questioning how, if porn, which has been so ubiquitous throughout their lives, is so sex-positive and liberating, why does the orgasm gap remain, with women significantly less likely to climax during a sexual encounter?[4] Cue all the responses saying an orgasm isn't everything (note this is being said to women, not men), as well as advice to women on how to fix the problem with articles on 'what women can do about it'.[5] And despite the pushback, these brave voices challenging the status quo are growing.[6] In a report on how many Gen Z women are disenchanted with living in a porn-saturated world, one woman lamented, 'It feels like we were tricked into exploiting ourselves [and] tricked into thinking it was our idea.'[7]

People are reluctant to agree that Big Porn is harmful. Not because it's a finely balanced argument, but because it's such a fraught subject, rooted in decades of controversy and heated debate. There's been so much misrepresentation of people's arguments, it's sometimes difficult to see through the abuse, deliberate misunderstandings and caricatures to what's really there. Too much heat and too little light.

It's also a challenge because I need to jump start a debate that is locked in the past. There's little acceptance that porn's role in society has dramatically changed due to the transformation of the porn industry (no longer a film industry in its own right) and its business model, which, as we saw in the last chapter, algorithmically dictates our viewing habits. Nor is there proper recognition that porn use is endemic. It's no longer niche, a pastime of a marginalised minority whose rights need protecting. Public discussions similarly remain dominated by those who grew up when a nude centrefold in *Playboy* was about as explicit as it got.

In addition, the resisters are focused on challenging 'censorship' by state bodies. But such arguments largely relate to an offline world where state-backed authorities regulated what was available in a sex shop. (They still do, but who gets their porn from a sex shop these days?) Most of these arguments fail to understand or acknowledge that it is Big Tech and Big Porn that are driving and controlling our choices, and in ways far beyond what even the most avid censor would ever manage to achieve. Unregulated and unaccountable private companies are deciding what we watch. It's Big Porn that now censors, using its heft to squash the creative side of the porn industry.

PARTICIPATORY PORN

Instead of futile arguments over cause and effect, more recent approaches to the harms of porn take a step back, considering behavioural changes more generally, as learned from the advertising industry. This is about the 'sexual scripts' that shape our lives.[8] The script of a play or film sets the scene and tells the story; a script is also a computer programme providing the sequence of instructions to be carried out. Sexual scripts are the narratives, meanings and messages whereby we ask and answer questions about sex: how do we know what sex is? What is everyone else doing? What is expected of us and others in sex? What might we want and like? What's normal? What's acceptable and what's not? What are the boundaries, if any?

Here's an example of how sexual scripts work. When researching mainstream porn in 2022, Elaine Craig came across the video 'my stepfather loves to fuck me without protection' on XHamster.[9] This video was offered following a search for 'wake-up' porn and showed a young woman first asleep and then trying repeatedly to resist the sexual advances of a male who eventually has sex with her. Now imagine a viewer, let's call him Man, comes across this video. Man gets his first indication of what the intended meaning of the video is from the title. If he clicks the link, he is choosing to watch a representation of sexual activity between a stepfather and his stepdaughter (it is tagged as amateur and homemade, encouraging Man to believe the content is real). Man can see that 80,000 others have already watched it. He is not alone. Of the thousands who have watched a depiction of a stepfather holding down his sleeping stepdaughter while he has sex with her, 99 percent gave it the thumbs up. Everyone else likes it, so it's OK to be sexually aroused by videos like these.

Man notices the video has been on the site for a few years; no one has reported it as portraying non-consensual sex or breaching any other terms of service – or if they have, their claim has been rejected. Man sees the tags for this video and suggestions of similar videos; he realises this is not just one random video, there's a whole genre of stepdaughter porn! In fact, it's a common category, not weird, perverted or out of the ordinary.

Finally, Man sees comments from other users saying things like 'good girl, fight it but take it after all' and 'my stepdaughter loved to fuck me'. Man now knows others found it arousing watching a depiction of a stepdaughter resisting but then acquiescing to sexual activity initiated while she was asleep. Man might not believe the commenter actually had sex with his stepdaughter, but he gets the message that he thought it worth making the comment – perhaps that was arousing itself – or he was hoping to ingratiate himself with others in the XHamster community.

This is how sexual scripting works. We get messages – titles, tags, users, the actors, where we find it, etc. – that mould our understanding of what sex is. This is how any media, including porn, shapes the sexual scripts that influence our intimate lives and our lives more generally. Man gets so many messages bolstering his desire to watch this type of material that, even if he were concerned at first, the messages erase any such qualms. There is no reckoning here that this is sexual assault, that it's not possible to consent to sexual activity when asleep. This is confirmed by the video having been there a while; it's permitted, and as the website terms of service clearly prohibit non-consensual material, this must be lawful. The video revels in gaining sexual arousal from a scene representing an older man having sex with a young woman whom he is supposed to protect and care for, affirmed by the videos shown alongside, which offer similar material.

Two years on from Craig analysing this video, it's still there; it's now been watched over one million times. Still no reports. Still all thumbs up and more approving comments. Next to it are videos clearly mimicking sexual activity with underage girls; they are wearing children's underwear and having sex on children's bedsheets. It's next to other videos labelled as women being asleep when sex is initiated, including a video titled 'waking up my stepdaughter with my big cock' – viewed 1.5 million times.

These are the sexual scripts shaping responses to the questions raised earlier, such as what is normal, what is expected and what is everyone else doing. This particular sexual script is saying it's acceptable to be aroused by sex with a sleeping family member and from videos suggesting sexual activity with underage girls. It reinforces that this is a common category of porn watched by millions. In watching, liking and commenting, you are part of a community of like-minded individuals.

XHamster has a community of over 50 million subscribers. It exemplifies the participatory nature of today's porn industry. Sexual scripts are not just about what's produced and pushed to us by porn platforms; they're informed by users too. In watching the video, clicking on the offered tags, in rating and commenting, we create new data, all logged by the porn platform and content creators, shaping future decisions about what content to make and offer us next. The platforms encourage us to comment and to create gifs and excerpts of our favourite videos to share online. Maybe some of the thousands of viewers of this video have shared their favourite part online, encouraging more to come and view it. Add algorithms into the mix, which push content towards us based on what we like, what we give thumbs up to, and these problematic sexual scripts become further normalised and reinforced.

Here we have a community of users egging each other on, normalising what is happening, validating their choices. This is not just a fantasy inside someone's head, passively watching then switching off. This is participatory porn, active engagement that produces new forms of porn that then exist in, and alter, our social worlds.[10]

Each seemingly small act collectively contributes to the sexual script, the social meaning applied to particular videos, which shapes the platform's algorithms. There's no secret in this. At the end of watching videos on XHamster, you get a pop-up encouraging you to rate the video 'to help our AI algorithm'. In doing so we are telling the algorithm not only that we watched it and liked it, but also that we did not flag it as problematic or in violation of the platform's terms of service. No need to worry, we can ignore those complaining about the porn industry. Therefore, while the community and users are actively contributing to the meaning of these videos, the porn platform is learning. Through data gathering and algorithms, the platform is shaping our values, attitudes and preferences; it is continually refining its product for maximum profit and consumption, and we happily play along.

In thinking about effects and harms, the question becomes, what is the impact of these particular sexual scripts? It raises so many questions and assumptions, such as: is that *really* sexual assault? Even if she didn't like it at first, she then seemed to, so is it rape? Or just 'wake-up sex'? She says she didn't consent, but how do we know, since women often seem to resist at first? Rather than the idea of sex with your young stepdaughter being abhorrent, it seems more common and acceptable than you might have thought. Maybe you don't do it (though maybe you do), but when others do, is it really so bad? Is she really so traumatised? So many of these girls seem precocious. Why spend so much public money on investigating cases of family abuse, or sexual assault when someone was sleeping, when it's not that serious or harmful? When young women complain about being leered at on public transport or in the streets, or by their father's friends, what do they expect? It's normal and just a bit of banter; they like it, really.

Some women will watch this stepdaughter video and doubt their own experiences: maybe I shouldn't feel uncomfortable when he starts having sex with me when I'm asleep. Maybe it's fine. Maybe I did something that made him think it was OK. Maybe I need to act differently. Men seem to take resistance as playing 'hard to get'. Maybe it's just normal for men to leer at me when I walk home from school. It seems like lots of my peers are having sex. I need to lighten up and not take this so seriously. What's the point in reporting my father's friend groping me, or my stepfather; who is going to believe me? The police say it will be difficult to prove; maybe they're right. My family and friends think it's not worth it. I don't want people to think I'm overreacting.

SCRIPTING OUR SEX LIVES

This idea of 'sexual scripts' was developed from research on how we all learn behaviours by observing others in real life and across all forms of mass media. Unless we think of our behaviours and sexual preferences as innate, biological, we learn them from somewhere. I don't think there is anything innately aggressive about male sexuality, or that incest is a natural and inevitable drive for a proportion of the population. This means behaviours can shift again, which is a cause for hope.

Therefore, the most basic position must be that exposure to pornography has some impact on its consumers, and that this prompts them to act in certain ways. In fact, due to its ubiquity, on these questions of sexual scripts it surely plays the leading role, especially as there is so little sex education or discussion about real sex – what it is, what we do, even what porn we use and what it means to us. It's largely consumed in silence, and we largely act in ignorance of what others are doing and thinking.

Put simply, porn doesn't exist in a silo, away from the reality of our lives, a pure, private fantasy divorced from any real-world impact. This is not to say that there's a direct, automatic process of taking information, such as porn, and then acting it out. However, it shapes how we think about sex, what we find appealing and what we see as acceptable sexual conduct.

Many nonetheless continue to claim that pornography has no effects beyond inducing orgasm. Yet this does not make sense when we consider how we assess the harm of any particular activity, advert or social media. Another way to think about this is in terms of probability, starting with the proposition that the probability of something being the case – such as the prevalence of sexual violence – is greater given its frequency in pornography than if it were not in pornography.[11] In other words, is it more likely that we continue to have high levels of sexual inequality and sexual violence, than if there was no such thing as patriarchal porn? My answer is: yes. More specifically, the reality of high levels of non-consensual sexual activity primarily against women and girls is more likely because of this type of porn.

This probability argument is common in all walks of life, including climate change and medicine. Just as no particular car, no particular factory, no particular individual failing to recycle directly causes climate change, the harms materialise from cumulative individual examples.[12] Similarly, we do not speak of a singular cause of problems such as lung cancer. We know what some of the key indicators are, what makes it more likely, but there are always cases that buck the trend. There are unfortunately those who have lung cancer and have never smoked, but if you continually smoke, you are far more likely to get lung cancer than if you don't.

Several factors typically work together, often reinforcing each other in a weblike causal mechanism. The same is true for heart disease.[13] While factors like obesity, high cholesterol, smoking, lack of exercise and so on can all lead to heart attacks, each one alone is likely insufficient, but that does not mean that they are not contributory factors to making heart disease more likely.

Therefore, just as we understand the harms of smoking in probabilistic terms, so we can say that mainstream porn is one key factor that actively raises the probability of harms, rather than being singly responsible for them. We can further say that it raises the likelihood quite significantly in view of the ubiquity of porn, the extreme nature of so much of it and its intensely eroticising format.

We also need to recognise that, in these debates over porn and its impacts, there are clear parallels with the strategies used to deny the harms of tobacco and now climate change.[14] Sceptics argue there is too much uncertainty, too much debate amongst the scientific community (often funded by large lobbies) to justify regulation. Sure, they say, there might be *some* possible harms, but at this time, there's not enough *direct evidence*, and so it's best just to watch and wait.

This claim to be ready to act if there were the right evidence is disingenuous, and yet it still dominates – and, crucially, stymies – debate. Those who defend pornography, or who challenge regulation, tend to deploy this argument about the need for evidence of *direct* causal effects, as they know that there is no definitive causal link. But what they do not go on to say is that there are no such studies because there never can be, nor ever will be. How would you design a study that controlled for any of the factors that influence sexually abusive behaviour? You can't, because the drivers of sexual violence are so complex and multifaceted that it is not possible to say that any one factor, including pornography, directly shapes a specific act.

It's not a question of monkey see, monkey do. It's the power of representations to shape what people desire and find attractive that insidiously, imperceptibly shapes our attitudes, our actions and our world. It's about probability, and the harms that are simply more likely because of this kind of porn.

It should be obvious. It's what Big Tech is all about. It's what the entire advertising and PR industries are all about. Sufficiently vivid, attractive and compelling representations can mould our appetites – that is, alter our sense of what is desirable or attractive.[15] After all, if adverts did not influence and make us do things we otherwise wouldn't, there would be no ad industry. The gambling industry, for example, has played a blinder, dominating many sports by mainstreaming gambling, normalising it and making it fashionable and cool. This shows the power of money, adverts and PR to manipulate attitudes, as well as to directly influence regulation (or rather the lack of). This is the world of mainstream porn, with its algorithms and business model and exceptionally effective marketing and political lobbying.

The sexual scripts of porn are commonly violent, misogynistic, racist and sexist, as well as propagating dangerous assumptions about young girls, incest and rape. They are minimising the harms of practices such as choking and strangulation and making us think that men's pleasure is rightly prioritised and that women enjoy sex where they get hurt, abused, dominated or persuaded into it. These sexually violent scripts influence the cultural context, the messaging, which normalises and justifies many forms of abuse and violence against women and girls. They shape the boundaries between appropriate and inappropriate sexual conduct through representations that stigmatise and criminalise some sexual behaviours, while instructing and encouraging others. They limit women's individual freedom to act, directly affecting the sexual lives and choices of women and girls. Overall, they perpetuate ideas of gendered inequality that adversely impact on all of us, women and men, boys and girls, whether we watch porn or not.

It is reasonable to conclude that this material is shaping society, influencing how we understand these phenomena. Do we take them seriously? Do we understand the harms? Does this blur the boundaries between what's lawful and what's not? Does this make light of serious harms? Does this encourage this activity by eroticising it? Does it make women, and some men, doubt their feelings of discomfort by repeatedly depicting an activity as routine or expected? This is about porn scripting our sexual activity, with impacts across all areas of life. When *Stylist* magazine asks whether porn is pressurising young women to expect physically aggressive sex, they're debating the sexual scripts shaping women's experiences.[16] For men too, while the privileging of their interests might seem like a win-win, when those interests are algorithmically designed, the lingering effects may not be so wanted or beneficial. They too begin to feel uncomfortable, yet drawn back again and again, the lure of a dopamine hit pulling them in. Pornography has become a cultural authority on sex and sexuality – it gets into our heads and it's difficult to get it out. This is nowhere more clear than in the lives of young people.

YOUNG PEOPLE: 'THE GIRLS IN PORN LIKE IT'

In 2023, the Children's Commissioner conducted research into young people's views on pornography. One girl talked about how her first boyfriend had been pulling her hair and 'yanking' her head back during sex. When she'd asked him about it, he said, 'I thought you might like it. The girls in porn like it.'[17] This echoes the response of another young woman, who put it frankly: 'porn is the starting point for young people when it comes to sex'.[18]

These experiences point us towards two concepts. First, that the practices common in Big Porn do not represent an authentic idea of what pleasurable sex might be like; boys are doing this not because it feels good, but because they've seen it in porn. Secondly, these boys are not inherently aggressive; it's not pre-ordained that they will engage in violent behaviours when experimenting with sex. This is what is presented to them as normal, expected and acceptable, and so, understandably, they take it up. We know young people try out what they see in porn; why wouldn't they?[19] Unless we believe that men and boys are inherently abusive, they must get their ideas and impetus for action from somewhere. And much of it is coming from mainstream, online porn.

Until very recently, teenagers had easy access to the largest porn sites for free on their smartphones, with boys and young men accessing porn more frequently, with one in five young men aged 16–21 viewing porn content at least once a day.[20] Girls are viewing porn because of its authority over their lives. We see this in the reasons young people give for seeking out pornography: it's about sexual gratification, as well as curiosity (everyone's talking about it), to 'learn' about sex, and pressure to 'fit in' with peers.[21]

Boys talk about how watching porn is a shared activity at school; they bond over it. Opting out is simply not realistic.

Because of the power and authority of porn, children are seeking it out at earlier and earlier ages. The average age in England that children first see pornography is thirteen, though 27 percent had seen it by age eleven and 10 percent by age nine.[22] The age of first viewing has other impacts, with those viewing porn by age eleven more likely to become frequent users.[23] Importantly, the more frequent viewers are those who have problematic understandings of consent and are more likely to engage in physically aggressive sex acts.[24] We don't yet know how effective the new age verification controls on pornography platforms will be, particularly as many teenagers are tech-savvy and manage to get around the controls.

Nonetheless, we still know that four out of five young people today have encountered violent pornography before the age of eighteen. Unsurprisingly, therefore, nearly half of young people said they thought girls enjoy physically aggressive sex acts, with just under half saying that boys expect sex to involve aggression.

Furthermore, there's a whole field of academic study that investigates what is referred to as 'problematic sexual behaviours' among teenagers, namely behaviours that are abusive, exploitative, aggressive and non-consensual. Overall, the research finds an association between pornography exposure and problematic sexual behaviours in teenage boys. One study involving over 16,000 children found significant associations between both violent and non-violent sexual content and harmful sexual behaviour.[25] Interestingly, while the risk increased with violent sexual content, it was not by a huge amount, with the researchers suggesting that mainstream porn contains enough degrading, objectifying and problematic material to be associated with increased sexual aggression.

This is echoed in another study, this time following teenagers over a number of years. It found higher levels of sexual violence associated with pornography use. In particular, non-violent pornography was associated with an almost three-fold increase in the odds of serious violence perpetration and violent pornography, and an almost four-fold increase in risk compared to no exposure to pornography over time.[26] As with all these studies, the authors are not saying that porn is the only cause of sexual violence or necessarily the most significant. This study further identified other risk factors, including alcohol and substance misuse, aggressive and delinquent behaviour, poor caregiver relations, behaviour problems at school and exposure to community violence. But, nonetheless, accessing violent pornography is a risk factor. Another way to think about all of these studies is that none of them observe reductions in problematic behaviour among young people exposed to porn. It's not beneficial, and it's not even neutral; it clearly increases the risks of perpetrating sexual violence. And young girls are the primary victims.

The adverse impacts are becoming more and more evident. In the UK, an increasing proportion of police reports of sexual assault and rape are of teenage boys offending against teenage girls, with some evidence of the influence of pornography in the behaviours of those being reported.[27] A few years ago, following serious revelations of the extent of sexual harassment and abuse in schools, Ofsted, the UK body responsible for maintaining school standards, reported that easy access to and high levels of pornography use was helping to normalise sexual abuse.[28] It talked of the 'warped' views of sex commonly found and 'deeply disturbing' approaches to consent. This is a pattern observed in many other countries too, where there are increasing reports of sexual violence being perpetrated by teenage boys against girls, with professionals identifying a clear relationship between the easy availability of violent pornography and a rise in harmful sexual behaviours.[29]

We need to face the reality of increasing numbers of young men perpetrating sexual violence against teenage girls, alongside studies reporting associations between porn use and problematic sexual behaviours. This cannot be ignored, dismissed as sex-negative or a 'moral panic', unless we are willing to ignore the distress and trauma experienced by so many young girls. It's not only acts of sexual violence that are increasing, but other forms of abuse, with evidence that higher pornography use is positively associated with image-based sexual abuse perpetration, such as sharing intimate images without consent.[30]

This is also impacting boys. Violence and aggression in sex is being encouraged and legitimised by porn and reinforced by the misogynistic content of male 'influencers'. But that doesn't mean that boys are the beneficiaries of porn culture. Instead they report feeling a pressure to perform, to look a certain way, to feel a certain way about sex. One young man explained that the 'real thing almost didn't turn me on enough', having watched so much porn when very young.[31] Many are saying they thought sex looked better in pornography than it was in real life.[32] Seriously, how disheartening is it that for young men (and likely even more for young women), sex in real life is *disappointing* because of porn? The impact goes beyond attitudes towards consent, or violence and abuse. It's about young people's developing sense of self, of relationships with others, of their mental and physical autonomy. Young people are growing up grappling with who they are, who they want to be, to share their own identities, feelings, sexualities; mainstream porn is hijacking their developing lives in multiple, harmful ways.

IT DOESN'T STOP AT EIGHTEEN

While there is an understandable focus on young people, the world does not suddenly change at age eighteen. Porn is still there, still shaping our sexual scripts. While women do watch pornography, men are far more frequent visitors of pornographic websites. The latest UK statistics found that, in May 2024, three-quarters of those accessing porn were men.[33]

The differences between women's and men's habits reveal the ways in which sexual preferences are diverging. Women are accessing erotic fiction sites such as Literotica, a site hosting erotic stories uploaded by users, as well as websites with erotic content targeting women.[34] Literotica can boast roughly 2.5 million registered users, and around 40 million visitors a month, 26 percent of these being women. In the UK, however, 45 percent of Literotica's 542,000 visitors are women. Nonetheless, this is a drop in the ocean compared to the ubiquity of Pornhub.

On mainstream sites, users aren't just watching porn. These are social networks, communities of the like-minded, exchanging messages and comments. The Pornhub community, commenting in their millions, is overwhelmingly male.[35] Unsurprisingly, when women are accessing Big Porn, it is often with considerable conflict due to its aggressive, misogynistic nature.[36]

Trying to work out the impact of these viewing habits has formed the basis of many studies over the years, often characterised as 'direct effects' debates. Many studies were conducted when porn was becoming increasingly accessible through the 1970s and 1980s, and when conflicts were growing between those characterising themselves as liberal and therefore open to all and any porn, and some feminists raising alarm at how it might be increasing violence against women and girls. These studies are limited in what they told us then, but particularly in what they offer us today.[37] For starters, what was labelled as hard-core or violent porn is relatively mild by today's standards. Some of these studies tried to test attitudes against a control group who hadn't watched porn – try finding such a group today!

What we do have today are studies that are trying to establish not direct cause and effect, but associations. A couple of years ago, researchers analysed 166 studies and found that exposure to pornography is positively associated with aggressive thoughts, attitudes and behaviours, and the link was stronger if the porn was violent.[38] Particularly interesting are the findings in relation to women, who rarely feature in these studies. Researchers discovered that viewing porn has similar effects, with women as susceptible as men to learning aggressive sexual scripts and developing aggressive thoughts, feelings, attitudes and behaviours towards other women.

This is why the sexual scripts of porn are pervasive and insidious on so many levels, encouraging women to accept aggressive behaviour and attitudes towards themselves, with the authors referring to this as women 'internalising oppression'.[39] Likewise, we can see this in recent projects investigating current attitudes and behaviours. In 2020, a study found that, among American adults of all ages, there is a statistically significant association between pornography use and engaging in rough sex behaviours, including what the authors somewhat ambiguously labelled 'penile-anal penetration without first asking/discussing', otherwise known as rape.[40] Similar results came from a study of university students from 2024, which found that those reporting higher pornography use were more likely to endorse risky sexual scripts, such as engaging in sex where consent was 'ambiguous'.[41]

Many analyses have uncovered how porn is exacerbating cultural misogyny. A report from the UK government in 2020 concluded that 'there is substantial evidence of an association between the use of pornography and harmful sexual attitudes and behaviours towards women'.[42] This included men having higher levels of acceptance of sexual aggression towards women and, for some, higher levels of perpetration of sexual aggression. The report further found that 'pornography use had a statistically significant association with attitudes supporting violence against women (with violent pornography showing an even stronger association)'.[43]

These studies only scratch the surface of the work that is being done on the impacts of pornography across society. Other research includes women reporting significantly less satisfaction with their bodies and their sexual lives where their male partners had higher porn use.[44] Similarly, the nature of mainstream porn is attributed by some to the lower rates of heterosexual sexual activity and relationship satisfaction, particularly among younger generations.[45] Men too are suffering, with phenomenal increases in young men experiencing erectile dysfunction, often associated with high porn use.[46] Some of this is related to performance anxiety and concerns over body image, as well as being connected to increases in what is called 'problematic porn use' amongst men.[47] From a public health perspective, Big Porn is wreaking havoc on our sexual lives.[48]

THE CULTURAL HARMS

Porn adversely shapes our cultural norms and attitudes, what my colleagues and I call 'cultural harm'.[49] By cultural harm, I mean it alters our sense of what's permissible and acceptable, and what crosses the line into sexual violence. Let's take the example of porn depicting sex without consent, an easily searchable and popular category. It clearly eroticises rape, making rape and other forms of sexual violence more likely by removing barriers to perpetration. It contributes to a culture that minimises the harms of rape, failing to take it seriously. This in turn leads to a society where, at the very least, rape is less likely to be recognised as rape (by police, prosecutors, judges and juries), where it is less likely to be investigated, where rape myths are harder to challenge. After all, how can an act that men regularly consume as an appealing 'fantasy' be really *that* bad?

We see this in research showing a strong link between frequent pornography use and acceptance of rape myths, such as 'she wanted it', 'he didn't really mean to' and 'it wasn't really rape'.[50] If women question whether what happened to them really was rape, they're less likely to report it or tell anyone else. Similarly, with attitudes towards deepfake sexual abuse – where a woman or girl's image is imposed into pornography without their consent – frequent users of pornography have been found to be far less bothered about this form of sexual harassment, perhaps due to becoming more immune to the abusive character of the material.[51]

However, the cultural harm of patriarchal porn extends beyond sustaining high levels of sexual violence. It perpetuates and glorifies gendered stereotypes. When investigating attitudes towards gender equality and sexism, studies have found that for both women and men there is a strong association between frequent pornography use and what is called benevolent sexism – seemingly positive or kind behaviours towards women, which in fact hold women back, rooted in stereotypes about women being less able than men.[52] Though hostile sexism – more directly discriminatory and negative – is stronger amongst men, the research tells us that both men and women are influenced by pornography. Sexism and gender inequalities are normalised and gender hierarchies are reinforced. Women are typically portrayed as passive, submissive or existing solely for male pleasure, while men must be bigger, stronger, more physical, more forceful and always up for sexual activity. These stereotypes reinforce sexual double standards celebrating men's sexual conquests while stigmatising women's sexual autonomy.

The cultural harm can be seen in the contribution to sexist, misogynistic attitudes and practices more generally, with cumulative impacts felt across society. We can see this in reports of misogyny in the police and other public services, with officers watching and sharing porn while on duty. There's the onslaught of sexualised and sometimes abusive commentary that often accompanies women's social media posts, as if women are just there as a target for men's banter, disdain and harassment. Sexual harassment is similarly sustained through the tropes of Big Porn. Girls talk about experiencing street harassment when in school uniform, connected to the prevalence of 'barely legal' and 'schoolgirl' porn and school uniforms being sold in sex shops.[53] One seventeen-year-old girl summed up her take on the impact of porn when she said that it quite simply 'makes boys act vile towards girls'.[54]

Big Porn also propagates deeply harmful stereotypes about racial and minority ethnic groups, reinforcing and eroticising colonialist and racist narratives. Legacies of slavery are evoked and sexualised, and representations of Asian people are reduced to stereotypes and fetishised. Black and minoritised young women talk about an unwelcome sexual curiosity from white men, evoked by porn.[55] 'They are going to try and go for me,' reported one young woman, 'because they have never had a Brown girl for it before, they are exotifying me.'[56] Some might argue it's possible to regularly watch porn with titles and tags like 'black slave' and 'black b*tch' (to include only what's printable) and be anti-racist in every other part of your life. I'm not convinced. Big Porn is reproducing racist language and stereotypes that would frankly be criminalised if published in any other media. Porn also commonly excludes or fetishises disabled individuals, and makes a mockery of the lives and experiences of LGBTQ+ individuals. Mainstream porn therefore is a form of cultural harm contributing to and sustaining structural inequality. It is damaging any sense of the importance of collective values around equality, liberty and freedom.

BIG PORN IS LIKE LEAD PAINT

To turn a question on its head, instead of asking, does porn cause harm? We can ask, where is the evidence that porn is *not* causing harm? What is the evidence that, unlike the whole advertising and PR industry, porn is somehow exempt from influencing our attitudes, desires and practices?

Many people have tried to come up with analogies to other harmful industries or products to try to explain the problem with porn. Some have said it's like tobacco, with a powerful industry that lobbied hard to convince us there was no harm. The problem with the tobacco analogy is that it leads you to prohibition, since it turns out smoking is never good for you and, as I argued in the Introduction, the problem is not with sexual expression itself but with the misogyny, sexual violence and racism of Big Porn.

Others have said it's like climate change and pollution. We can't say that a particular storm or flood is the result of climate change, but we can say that it changes the odds, making it more likely. It's not one individual act that causes pollution or climate change, but the accumulation of individual decisions and behaviours. (Pornhub responded to this analogy by filming a porn movie on a plastic-infested beach, titled the 'dirtiest porn ever'. Now, when you search 'porn and pollution', you see a wave of good PR for Pornhub.)

I think the more convincing analogy is that patriarchal porn is like lead in paint.[57] It may seem vital at first, useful even. Then we realise, slowly, that it's seriously harmful, a silent killer. But the resistance against change is strong from those used to the supposed benefits, as well as the companies producing it. Eventually though, non-toxic paint is developed, and in time we wonder what on earth all the fuss was about, and why we resisted change for so long.

In many walks of life, health and climate change being just two, an approach to considering harm based on probability and wider societal level impacts is entirely accepted, and to think otherwise, especially in a medical context, would be quite bizarre. Yet, in relation to pornography, it seems there is such societal reluctance to accept the obvious. Challenging the dominance of the pro-porn, right to porn, porn as sex-positive narrative leaves many of us facing harassment, abuse and accusations of moral puritanism or religious fanaticism. I actually do think of myself as sex-positive. And it's precisely because of this that I think we need to regulate porn, so we can begin to build a society that truly values women's sexual pleasure.

Big Porn has a direct, adverse impact on individual women and girls, limiting our freedom and liberty. It creates the cultural conditions for sexual violence, with the boundaries between what is lawful and what is not, what is acceptable and what is not, being rendered unclear. Overall, it is perpetuating ideas of gendered inequality that adversely impact on all of us, women and men, girls and boys, whether we watch porn regularly or never. Our sexuality, our sense of self, our values are being manipulated by an industry designed for maximum profit.

It's up to us to demand non-toxic sexual content: porn without the patriarchy. This is not about limiting sexual freedom and liberty, or banning sex or porn. It's about genuine liberation, which requires reform and regulation. But before we get to that, let's look at the pornographic scenarios being played out in Big Porn.

3

Rough

I HAVE A DISUSED COMPUTER SITTING IN THE CORNER OF MY university office. It looks like it should be in the Design Museum. It's got ports for CDs and DVDs and is infuriatingly slow. You switch it on, get a cup of coffee, and then it might just be ready to go. It's the Porn Computer: the computer dedicated to the specific task of uncovering what the most popular mainstream porn sites offer to first-time viewers, mostly young teenage boys. I conducted this research a few years ago with my colleague, Fiona Vera-Gray, and it's one of the largest studies of online porn content. We wanted to find out what was on the most popular porn websites, and we needed a dedicated computer. Not a nice new one; that would be a waste. We were given an ancient computer that could be cast aside after its memory had been filled with porn. And the computer has ended its life corrupted by porn. It's still in my office, in front of me each day, as I can't face the bureaucracy necessary to get it removed and decommissioned. Maybe one day, someone will recover the hard drive and wonder how on earth this porn was allowed to be so freely and easily accessible.

All of this – the designated computer equipment, the exceptional ethics approval, even meetings with the local police – was for a study looking into the material that millions are accessing on their phones, laptops and computers every minute of every day. The porn we were viewing was not on the dark web; it was the porn that shapes all our lives. Yet we could only officially study it in this very constrained way. In some ways, that was a good thing. Then, as now, watching this porn is debilitating, inducing despair and anger in equal measure. Watching it only on a specific computer, in the workplace, provided some guardrails.

So what did we find? We collected a database of over 150,000 videos and found that one in eight titles of the videos on the front page of the three most popular pornography websites described acts of sexual violence. This is what the porn platforms were choosing to showcase to new users: not what people were searching for, but what was being presented in their 'shop window'. Although staggering, this figure was conservative. We excluded anything advertised as part of BDSM practices or including terms associated with those acts, and we did not include verbal aggression such as 'dumb slut gets fucked' or 'come to Daddy bitch'. As our focus was on what could be defined as sexual violence, we excluded degrading and humiliating material such as 'daddy piss and spit' or 'Fuck me like you hate me'.

Our study has had an enormous impact, being used across the world to explain the extent of sexually violent material online. It's helped shape campaigns, law reforms and educational materials. It's cited in United Nations documents, government reports, Parliamentary speeches and newspaper columns in different countries. The impact of the work lives on in us as researchers. It made me realise how much had shifted with the business model of Big Porn and the ease of access of the internet.

'ROUGH SEX' IS JUST SEX

I'll start with 'rough sex', a term that covers a wide range of behaviours.[1] It includes acts that are forms of sexual assault, such as 'making someone have sex' (as the research studies describe it), as well as behaviours like hitting, spitting, pissing, pushing, hair-pulling, punching, biting, gagging, choking/strangulation and slapping. It can include acts that might be described as rough, depending on the context, such as 'hard thrusting' or 'being pinned down'.[2] Rough sex in porn is about the ways in which many sexual acts are performed, often involving verbally aggressive or derogatory language and predominantly performed by men against women. Sometimes women are shown liking the rough acts, sometimes they are shown in clear distress. There's a lot of this material in porn. Rough sex is so normalised and common that it's rarely labelled as such, making it difficult to quantify.[3]

It's the mundanity of rough sex that makes any discussion tricky. That's because, for many younger people, rough sex *is* sex.[4] At a recent event discussing rough sex and sexual violence, I realised that, when speaking to some young women, they were using the same words as me but speaking a different language. When I hear the phrase 'rough sex', I hear 'rough' and understand rough sex as distinct from sex. But for them, they do not hear the word rough; it is just sex.[5] Rough sex is what sex is, not because it's preferred but because they assume that's all there is. My response was: er, no. That while there has always been some aggression in some sex and porn, the mainstreaming of rough sex as a thing (and supposedly a good thing) is a far more recent cultural phenomenon, and there are *so* many other ways to be having sex.

It's not possible to map a direct timeline, but over the last ten to fifteen years we can chart the popularising of 'rough sex', from a label describing particularly extreme practices and violent acts on the periphery to a conventional, acceptable and legitimate form of sexual practice.[6] It's now masquerading as synonymous with sex and is a dominant part of porn. A recent study with young people aged 16–21 found that nearly half thought girls 'expect' sex to involve physical aggression, and a further 42 percent stated that most girls 'enjoy' acts of sexual aggression.[7]

Now, if this was just about changing sexual habits or attitudes, it would be interesting, but not necessarily problematic. However, there is a darker underbelly to this change, and it's one that young women particularly have been raising, although they often don't have the words to describe it. As rough sex has been normalised, many women have spoken about their own troubled relationship with these practices. Rachel Thompson wrote the powerful book *Rough* about how 'violence has found its way into the bedroom'.[8] She shares the experiences of women who didn't have the words to define what happened to them, who experienced behaviours that didn't match what they consented to, or felt it must be a 'grey area' or 'not rape but …' These are women who were harmed but didn't believe they had the right to feel aggrieved.[9]

This sense of unease comes out of research with women about their experiences of rough sex that are unexpected and not pleasurable, but accepted as consensual.[10] Yet there's a sense of something being not quite right, the experience being one of sexual compliance, rather than something wanted or enjoyed. Some of this dissonance comes from women's sense of expectations around what is normal, expected and what they are supposed to want. Young women sometimes describe their sexual partners being kind and loving after some of these unnerving and exploitative experiences, and that they want relationships with the men acting in these abusive ways towards them.[11]

Some of these young men may have little idea that their behaviours are so unsettling and uncomfortable because they too think this is normal, just sex. In one recent survey, a third of men reported they wouldn't seek consent from a partner before engaging in rough sex. This is both disturbing and entirely understandable. Asked what prompted the men to slap, choke, spit on or gag their partner (nearly three-quarters said they'd done these acts), just over half said porn, with one fifth saying this had influenced them a 'great deal'.[12] This is similar to other studies finding that watching rough porn is positively associated with desire for and participation in rough sex.[13] I will return to these issues, to what all of this might mean for choice, consent and women's sexual pleasure, but first we need to consider in a bit more detail what is in patriarchal porn and what is it telling us about sex and aggression.

AGGRESSION IN PORN

Let's start with the research into the extent of physical or verbal aggression, which overall has found that a substantial amount of porn, at least half of mainstream videos and probably more, includes aggression, mostly physical aggression.[14] But these content analyses struggle with definitions. For example, one commonly quoted study from 2010 included any physically aggressive acts whether the target expressed pleasure, displeasure or was neutral.[15] It found that 88 percent of porn included aggression. Alternatively, other researchers have only counted material as aggressive if the target clearly conveyed that they did not want to participate and were then forced. Seeing as women in porn are generally shown to enjoy anything and everything, not surprisingly, that study yielded the very low figure of 2 percent of content being aggressive.[16] Most studies land somewhere in between, hence why saying that overall, perhaps about half of all mainstream porn includes physical aggression.

The studies include acts like pushing, pulling, slapping, choking, strangulation, gagging, punching, biting, spitting, spanking, restraining or holding down forcefully, hair-pulling, forced sex and similar as physical aggression. Verbal aggression involves derogatory or demeaning language. Interestingly, what's not covered in these studies is psychological aggression in the form of coercion and exploitation.

The amount of aggression and how it is marketed varies across different genres, with aggressive behaviours more readily advertised in titles for the 'teen' category.[17] We see this in titles such as 'Extra Small Teen Fucked To Her Limit In Extreme Rough Sex Session', which has 15 million views. Porn involving Black and minoritised people is often more aggressive. Just in case it's not clear, another study calculated that women were the target of the aggression in 97 percent of scenes, men the aggressors in 76 percent and the women's responses to aggression were nearly always neutral or positive.[18]

These researchers all analysed the videos themselves, whereas my content study focused on the video titles, going beyond the specifics of the acts, telling us something more disturbing – what it all means. A title suggests to you how you might understand the video. Pornhub knows the value of titles, informing those uploading videos that 'Rather than stating "what" they will see, use the title to describe "how" they will see it.'[19]

Large numbers of the titles we categorised as aggression included words like abuse, ambush, break, brutal, destroy, drill, pain, ram, slam, pound, punish, torture, with fewer including stab, assault, victim, punch and even a few managed to spell annihilate. These terms convey so much more than the naming of a specific act, or even a category such as 'rough sex'. They give a far greater sense of what is really out there, such as 'extreme brutal face fucking for this bound helpless slut! But she loves it!' This title tells us that, at some level, there is surprise – the exclamation mark – that women do supposedly 'enjoy' this. These titles insult the woman and revel in her humiliation.

HOW PORN TURNED SPITTING INTO SEX

Beyond the more obvious forms of physical aggression, there are other acts that can fall within the scope of rough sex, including spitting. How common do you think this is? Your answer possibly varies depending on your age. When I read a recent survey finding that one in five young women had experienced spitting, I was shocked.[20] I thought this frequency was really high for a disturbing practice. Since then, however, I've come to learn that many young women think this figure is a huge under-estimate. They say it is commonplace. To say that it's unwanted or gross would be to stand out, to go against the grain, to be labelled vanilla, i.e. uncool.

Many practices come under the label 'spitting', with kissing of course also including the exchange of saliva. Nonetheless, this is another shifting norm: even if spitting in everyday life is understood as aggressive and humiliating, we're now supposed to accept it as a normal and acceptable part of ordinary sex and porn. It's successfully been given its own supposedly progressive label, 'spit kink'.[21] Spitting is part of many different sexual scenarios, but as part of rough, aggressive sex, it's very popular. Titles such as 'Spit covered blonde likes rough sex' had been watched 3.9 million times when I visited XVideos recently, though that's nothing like as popular as 'Facial destruction! Non-stop face-fucking rough gagging and extreme messy cum and spit drooling', which had nearly 12 million hits.

This seems to be another example of a powerful disconnect between everyday life and porn. To be spat on, even by a loved one, would usually be understood automatically as offensive, humiliating and aggressive. Think of two men outside the pub late at night sizing each other up. One spits on the other. The man spat on doesn't say: ooh that's lovely, do it again. He knows it's aggressive. He knows it's a power play. The police are likely to be on their way soon to deal with the fall-out. You can be prosecuted for spitting on someone without their consent, whether as part of sex or not; it's an assault.

But in porn and sex, women have been acculturated into accepting it as sexy. It might be arousing for him, but why? Because of power, humiliation and domination? Because he's able to act out what he's seen in porn? Some will say that's what BDSM is about, and maybe that's true, but that's niche, and a very particular practice. This is something much more common. We see it across social media, with some men talking about it in a clearly aggressive, dominant way, such as one influencer on TikTok saying 'I was with this girl, and I was on top, hand around her throat, and I looked down and said "open your fucking mouth" and she did. And I spat in her mouth.'[22] And he loved it. A woman influencer on Instagram challenged this man and his video, pointing out a lack of consent, and she faced a furious backlash. That dreaded label 'sex-negative' is applied to shut us all down.

I'm not criticising or 'kink-shaming' women who want to be spat on or want to spit on others. I know that, as well as the men bragging about their sexual activities, there are women declaring they'd let a particular man or celebrity spit on them, as an indication of their desire for them. (There's an alternative reading of this trend, of course: that someone is so attractive that they are worth suffering otherwise distasteful activities.)

The elephant in this bedroom is the misogyny in the air we breathe convincing us that what is happening is acceptable, progressive even. Things are being done to women, often as a powerplay, often deliberately belittling; it's the eroticisation of gendered inequality. We are quite plainly being convinced – through the porn algorithm replicated thousands of times over and seeping into sexual practices – that a practice that in every other context would be clearly understood as humiliating and unacceptable is something we should welcome. Conversations are shut down; the rhetoric of sex-positivity, no matter what, dominates. Patriarchy in action.

ROUGH SEX, CONSENT AND PATRIARCHY

The cultural dominance of rough sex and rough porn has particularly serious consequences when it's invoked as a defence by men who kill women during sexual activity. Acts that would once have been recognised as violent and showing a real intention to harm and kill are now given an 'air of reality'; the men have 'plausible deniability' by relying on a defence of 'rough sex gone wrong'.[23] This is a serious and growing problem in the UK and around the world, with the number of men relying on this defence increasing considerably in recent years.[24]

The issue came to particular prominence a few years ago, when British student Grace Millane was murdered while travelling in New Zealand, by a man using this argument.[25] The defence – and news reports around the world – continually referred to 'rough sex', 'kinks', 'erotic asphyxiation', 'pressure to the neck', 'powerplay', and more, all normalising and sanitising his actions. The jury didn't accept the defence and convicted the defendant of murder, but the cultural messages and headlines live on. Many juries in such cases do believe defendants, convicting of manslaughter rather than murder, or acquitting entirely, and many more cases don't even get before a jury because the chances of conviction are so low in light of the believability of the defence.

As discovered during my discussions with young women, rough sex for many *is* sex, which may explain the lack of discussions around consent between sexual partners. In a sexual culture dominated by mainstream porn, we are convinced this is what we want (because what else is there?). We're being persuaded into framing women's pain or discomfort as something to be enjoyed or ignored, by women and men.

But the language of consent does not magic away the problems of how some young women are experiencing rough sex. Many women say they consent but sometimes feel disturbed, having a sense of unease. They're not describing what happens to them as sexual assault (though it would commonly meet a legal definition). They are accepting it, complying with sexual norms. Not everyone, but many do.

Some men may feel similarly perturbed, a sense of dread over the expectation to behave a certain way. Nonetheless, that likely manifests in different ways, as they are the more empowered in these scenarios. They are the one whose sexual entitlement and sexual pleasure is privileged and valorised. They have been encouraged through this type of porn to prioritise their needs, wants and desires, not even thinking about, or deliberately ignoring, the interests of their partners.

Remembering the business model of Big Porn, we might ask: is spitting, pissing or gagging until your eyes water and mascara runs down your face authentic desire or algorithmic desire? In a world shaped by porn, women's pleasure and sexual autonomy seemingly isn't as desirable as a women's humiliation. This encourages (very successfully) a way of doing and thinking about sex that sanctions aggression against women.

Ultimately, I'm trying to separate the 'rough' from the 'sex', asking what are young women, in particular, missing out on? I want more questions to be asked about other ways of having sex, of being sexual, reminding us that this porn is not a world where women are having the time of their sexual lives. The prominence of words such as 'gets' in titles confirms this: porn sex is something done to the woman or young girl. There's no pretence of mutuality. Of course, porn is not causing or driving this on its own. Rough sex is a cultural phenomenon depicted in contemporary films, novels and social media. But porn is playing a defining role.

THE POWER OF FACIALS

Then there's practices like facial ejaculation, which are sometimes part of 'rough sex', sometimes not, and are often referred to as a 'cum shot', the 'money shot' or, commonly, just a 'facial'. Yes, when some people mention facials, they might not be talking about a beauty practice. It seems porn producers feel the need to convey that the action has finished, so you know the man has reached his heights of ecstasy (who cares about the woman), just in case you hadn't realised. But this doesn't just happen in porn; it's normalised in sexual practices today, and often in ways that are not welcome.[26] Younger women report that this happens in sexual encounters without their consent, like it's just part of what sex is.

There is little doubt that this practice dominates sexual culture due to porn. Sure, it predates video. The delightful Marquis de Sade wrote: 'I squirt the fuck in their face ... that's my passion.'[27] However, it was with the 1970s porn film *Deep Throat*, supposedly the highest-grossing porn film of all time[28] (as well as being an actual depiction of the rape and coercion of the main star, Linda Boreman), that the 'cum shot' became embedded in porn culture.

The point is not that facial ejaculation is always unwanted (though when we talk about it being wanted, we have to ask ourselves what this means in a sexual culture saturated by porn). But it is problematic that it has become so normalised, that it's assumed to be acceptable, when many women do not want it. Many talk about it being humiliating, an exercise of power and control. Some men have said they found facial ejaculation in pornography strange and repulsive at first, but after repeated viewing they began to think of it as normal and expected.[29]

Then there are men who explain they wouldn't do it with their girlfriends, as they 'respect them', but it's OK with hook-ups or women one man referred to as 'scumbags'.[30] This begins to lift the lid on this practice, revealing that it's often a powerplay, and that some men want to act out what they see, replicating videos with titles such as 'extreme facial abuse'. There's further evidence of this being a powerplay, with one study finding that teens were about five times more likely to feature in videos where the male performer ejaculated in their mouth or on their face.[31]

Facial ejaculation is related to what some call 'cum tributes', where a man ejaculates onto a woman's photo and posts it online without her consent. The images chosen are often from social media, and women in the public eye are commonly targeted.[32] There are vast numbers of online forums, as well as websites and private online spaces, entirely dedicated to these semen images, one of which received 4.8 million visits a month in 2022.[33] While the language of tributes is used, these are anything but: 'I hate all these women' reads one comment.[34] Another says, 'I want to see them degraded into sperm-covered rags.'[35] This is why the label 'hatewank' is far more apt than anything resembling a tribute.[36] Unfortunately, but not surprisingly, there is also a whole host of racist material, with videos on one of the main sites being tagged 'racist hatewank'.

While this hatewank material is deeply disturbing, I recognise that there are women embracing facials, such as in many profiles on X, from those inviting 'tributes' as part of their marketing for their sex work. My critique is not about them. They are trying to do what they can in this world propped up by Big Porn.

TALKING ABOUT ANAL SEX

I wasn't going to write about anal sex. I obviously knew that as a sexual practice it's become increasingly mainstream.[37] I knew many have been saying for years this is due to its promotion in porn, with porn actors and producers themselves acknowledging this. I knew from my own research that one in five of all the aggressive titles we found on the most popular porn sites included the words 'ass' or 'anal', suggesting a connection between physical aggression and anal sex. This will not come as a surprise to anyone who takes a brief look at the titles of videos online, such as 'unexpected anal' or 'it hurts anal'. This phenomenon even has its own word – 'painal' – alongside the oh-so-witty titles such as 'oops should've used lube'. Without properly questioning myself, I didn't want to go there, to where the backlash, the chant of 'kink-shaming' would be so loud. I'd internalised the normalisation of it.

This changed in late 2024, when I participated in a Parliamentary roundtable on pornography at which Louise Barraclough spoke. Louise has worked for decades in sexual health and has been the safeguarding lead for Devon and Cornwall sexual assault referral centres for many years. She didn't shy away from her subject, talking very clearly about the increased rates of faecal incontinence and anal sphincter injury in women who have anal sex. What I didn't realise, to my shame, is that women are at a higher risk of incontinence following anal sex than men, because of their different anatomy and the effects of hormones, pregnancy and childbirth on the pelvic floor. Louise referred to a *British Medical Journal* editorial talking about how women have less robust anal sphincters and lower anal canal pressures than men, and damage caused by anal penetration is therefore more consequential.[38] So it's not only that sexual scripts in porn commonly associate anal sex with pain and coercion, encouraging acting without protections such as lubrication, but that, due to women's different anatomies, this is simply far more risky and potentially harmful for them than vaginal penetration.

But this reality and risk of harm is not widely known, and hardly anyone is talking about it. There is indeed a fear or a lack of courage – such as I had – to raise it. The NHS website just discusses the risk of sexually transmitted infections (STIs), with other media much the same. We are letting down a generation of young women by not talking about its significant risks beyond STIs. As Louise so movingly said, the prevalence of anal sex in porn is normalising harmful practices, without any counter-narrative informing women of the realities, the health risks and the ways they could protect themselves.[39] A better public discussion would empower those who are feeling pressured into anal sex.

'HIDDEN CAM CAUGHT GIRL ON TOILET'

Another area where the boundaries of consent and legitimacy are being challenged is the category of content that can be labelled 'image-based sexual abuse', where nude or sexual images are being created, solicited, taken and shared online without consent. A lot of this non-consensual material is uploaded to porn sites. It's a way to incur maximum humiliation and violation: millions can view the material; it spreads like wildfire, becoming almost impossible to remove from the internet. There are many lawsuits against Pornhub going through the courts that relate to all manner of non-consensual material, including recordings of sexual assaults and rapes that were shared on Pornhub and which they failed to take down for many years.[40] So many women's lives have been devastated by the pain and rupture resulting from their most private and intimate images being shared online without their consent; it's been life-ending for some, life-shattering for many others.

A few years ago, I spoke to Anna, whose ex-partner shared sexual videos of her online without her consent.[41] She told me that, when she found out what he'd done, her 'whole world just crumbled'. She completely withdrew from life, knowing so many in her community had seen the videos shared widely online. In an attempt not to be identified, she drastically altered her weight, her hair. It was 'hell on earth' and never-ending, with videos continuing to circulate no matter how many times she tried to get them taken down. The police didn't care; the platforms didn't care. She worried about having to tell her children one day soon, before others in their class did. She had a breakdown and tried to kill herself. She described the whole experience as 'torture for the soul'.[42]

Anna is one woman, but her experiences resonate with many. My afternoon with Anna deeply affected me, even though I'd spoken with many survivors through my work. She expressed so well the whole-body, whole-person social rupture of this harm, affecting every aspect of her life, and it affected me so much because this was not being taken seriously by society – and it still isn't. She even felt the burden to try to make me feel alright about it all, trying to convince me she was now managing. I hope she is.

Anna's story formed part of my research with colleagues on women's experiences of image-based sexual abuse, research helping to shift the attitudes that minimise the harms experienced. I put Anna in touch with a journalist who faithfully reported her story, reaching a wide audience, hopefully giving comfort to some who saw Anna's story reflected in their own.[43]

I share Anna's experiences here to ensure we have her in mind when we consider the ease with which this material is spread online, the recalcitrance of platforms and social media to remove it swiftly, and the role of mainstream porn in trivialising and normalising this abuse.

My content study was the first to examine this particular type of material in Big Porn. We found it to be a common category, particularly voyeuristic videos involving hidden cameras and spy cams, and described using terms such as 'leaked', 'peeping' and 'private'. We're not saying that the titles are describing videos that were actually made and/or distributed without the consent of those featured (many will be representations), but we don't know, and some look suspiciously real.

Rather, our study shows how image-based sexual abuse is presented as a legitimate practice, a reasonable sexual fantasy. We found a predominant focus on voyeurism, both explicitly and through more implicit terms like 'hidden' or 'spy cameras', such as 'Beach Spy Changing Room Two Girls' and 'Japanese schoolgirl upskirt and downblouse' and 'hidden spycam doctor exam'. There was a lot of material about upskirting, such as 'Upskirted in the train'. A recent study of mainstream porn found voyeuristic material to be common, with terms 'cam videos', 'real hidden camera' and 'voyeur' among the most popular video tags.[44] Indeed, on XVideos, 5.7 million have watched 'Amateur blonde has no idea about spy cams'.[45]

This genre of porn legitimises non-consensual sexual acts. It sends a clear message that it's OK to gain sexual gratification from scenarios violating privacy, glorifying non-consent and abuse. There's no pretence here, no ambiguity; terms like 'hidden cam' clearly involve a lack of consent. We don't seem to realise that men perpetrating acts of voyeurism are among some of the more dangerous sexual offenders, yet they can go onto Big Porn and see millions gaining sexual arousal from the acts that they perform (and maybe videos they share). What are they to make of that? That it's acceptable? Of course, there is a difference between watching and perpetration. But we are failing to see that the voyeurism offender is encouraged in his acts (and in the knowledge that he's so unlikely ever to be prosecuted or convicted) by a culture tolerant of this conduct, and monetising it on the internet. Tiny changes are being made; Pornhub does block a search for 'hidden cam'. But, as with most of the material I discuss, it's still findable. Type 'hidden cam and Pornhub' into Google and it takes you to Pornhub pages labelled not 'hidden cam' but 'hidden real cam' or 'hidden sex cam'. Not a huge difference. Having said that, other sites like XVideos have not even taken this tiny baby step.

Once again, women's non-consent is being celebrated, enjoyed, sought out for sexual arousal. Some steps have been taken to reduce the amount of real abuse material on some of the porn sites, though not enough is being done. In any case, those changes are thoroughly undermined by the continued prevalence of material reproducing image-based sexual abuse. Anna and others like her will continue to experience 'torture for the soul' until we stop minimising non-consent and normalising it as a legitimate sexual fantasy widely available in porn.

EXPLOITATION AS ENTERTAINMENT

Some say that sexual fantasy is commonly based on eroticising power imbalances. Perhaps that's true. But I don't think that gives

Big Porn a free pass when it comes to minimising and legitimising forms of coercion and exploitation. I'm not talking about the material found in the aggression studies, or the clear representations of non-consent already examined in this chapter. What I mean are the videos that blur the boundaries between consent and non-consent. This is a discussion about scenarios that, at one level, are willingly undertaken, but – all things being equal – there really would be no agreement to this sexual activity.

Take the examples where cash is in a title, such as 'Chubby Spanish Teen Needs The Cash'. This is about gaining sexual arousal from a scenario where you know the other person is desperate, not for sex with you, but for money; and as you are able to give them money, on your terms, you feel powerful. Taken in isolation, as one random video, this might not seem too problematic. But there is a broader social and political context, namely that in Big Porn (as in society) this is mostly (older) men with power, abusing that power to gain sex with women who have few options. Social inequality has been made erotic; exploitation has been made desirable.

There are multiple examples of sex in law enforcement settings, such as the blatant 'police takes advantage of young girl to fuck her ass', as well as a whole genre of shoplifting videos where the male officer exercises power over young women and girls. In my content study, we found that the top three most common words in this category of coercion and exploitation all highlighted the youth of performers: schoolgirl, girl and teen. Many of these scenarios also involve Black and minoritised women. There are very popular genres involving war and migration, such as 'border controls', and when Russia invaded Ukraine in 2022, there was a 300 percent increase in online searches for 'Ukrainian refugee porn' and 'Ukrainian rape'.[46]

I'm not saying this material should all be unlawful. But I would like us to stop and think about it more, about its prevalence, about what messages this conveys, about who is using it, who is pushing this to us, why we are viewing this material and what it means for us all as a society.

WHAT ABOUT WOMEN'S SEXUAL PLEASURE?

While most of this book is focusing on the increasingly extreme nature of mainstream porn, I hope this chapter has conveyed some sense of the broader context, the supposedly more tame or less problematic material. Yet even this porn should be concerning, with its clear misogyny and racism, and the seemingly common desire to humiliate and punish women. It's this material that lays the foundations and sets the tone for how sex is understood and how women are treated in porn.

So while we may focus on the extremes, as I do throughout the majority of this book, it does not mean that the other material is OK. Spitting, facials, rough sex, coercion and exploitation, most of this sits on the boundaries of consent. Indeed, a major concern with mainstream porn is that it (deliberately) blurs notions of consent. However, even consent is not the ultimate standard. It is necessary, but it is not sufficient for us to have pleasurable, welcome sex. Another way to think of consent is as a floor, not the ceiling, for our expectations.[47] Consent is agreement to sex – it must not be conflated with desire, enjoyment or enthusiasm. I can consent to having my teeth drilled, but I don't welcome it and – all things considered – I wish I really didn't have to get it done.

It's likely my arguments will be challenged by those who will say many enjoy a powerplay and that probably holds some truth. They will further say that viewers will appreciate videos in different ways. That's true, and if we were talking about niche, pay-per-view sites with this material, I would be having a different conversation. But we're not. This is mass-produced porn for profit, algorithmically fed to us in our millions.

And the one thing this megalithic and monolithic porn is not about is women's sexual pleasure. In true academic understatement, scientific studies refer to this as 'orgasm inequalities' that are 'universally observed' in porn.[48] We also see this when women report lower satisfaction in their sexual relationships compared to men, and that while 'good sex' for men means orgasm, for women it's simply an absence of pain.[49] Mainstream porn, in all its guises, is stifling our sexual imagination, not even open to investigating or celebrating women's sexual pleasure. Here we are, decades into an experiment of the effects of easy, free and ubiquitous porn, and there is little evidence yet of 'sex-positivity' having much meaning in the lives of so many women and girls.

This is not about requiring individual women to get better at demanding consent or demanding what they want. This is societal; it's about inequalities of access to pleasure, desire, voice. Mainstream porn is silencing alternative sexual scripts, ones that valorise women's pleasure, speak to their desires and grant them meaningful power in sexual encounters. This isn't an issue confined to the bedroom; it's a political issue. Extreme porn is big business, one that governments have so far shown little interest in regulating. And that's precisely because our society prioritises, at every level, male pleasure over women's rights.

Big Porn is the pinnacle of patriarchy. It lacks any nuance in its message of men's pleasure being more important, privileging men's entitlement to sex whenever, with whomever and however they want. No matter how much we drape this in an empowering 'sex-positive' narrative of a brand-new era of sexual freedom, where there is no stigma or shame in any act, we can't blind ourselves to the reality. A world in which the most popular porn promotes women being dominated, coerced and violated does not have women's interests in mind.

4

Colour Coded

Racism thrives in porn. The abundant use of racist language and racist stereotypes would receive widespread condemnation in any other form of media. Yet somehow, as with eroticising violence against women and girls, porn gets a free pass, minimised as 'race play'. Millions watch it; millions scroll past it; it's become a cultural and political backdrop to our lives. But in the face of explicit and repeated racism, we encounter silence and denial.[1]

In this chapter, I share some of the ways that racist stereotypes are reproduced in Big Porn, particularly the more aggressive nature of porn involving Black men and women. I discuss the stereotypes of Asian women and the disturbing rise of 'hijab' porn. While racism infects all categories of porn, and must not just be examined in isolation, it is valuable to spend some time identifying its particularly insidious nature. We ought to consider the ripple effects, such as AI being trained on the aggressive and stereotyped associations of Black and minoritised women in pornography.[2] To borrow Audre Lorde's concept, what we are living with is 'racist patriarchy' in action.[3]

As with other areas of Big Porn, this is a complicated topic. For example, I will talk about how some women report positive experiences where porn shows Black women as sexually desirable. It is delicate navigating a path between the need to reduce racism and the risk of erasing race from its potentially positive representative ability to shape sexual scripts in progressive ways. Terminology raises complex issues. I follow the practice of organisations working to end racism by referring to Black and minoritised communities, as well as racialised communities.[4]

SLAVERY-ERA SEXUAL IDEOLOGIES

The racist tropes in mainstream porn arise from histories of slavery, colonialism and the ways in which Black men and women's bodies were paraded, objectified and mutilated. Writer Afua Hirsch refers to this as the legacy of 'slavery-era sexual ideologies' which are exhibited and reproduced in porn.[5] Not surprisingly, the racism in porn has been the target of criticism by some of the most celebrated Black women writers of our times. Patricia Hill Collins draws attention to the portrayal of Black women in pornography and its relationship with their historical and current inequality. She argues that the racism in pornography sexualises racist oppression, replicating hierarchies among women by drawing on a white supremacist history of exploiting Black women's bodies.[6] Just as gender inequality and misogyny is eroticised in Big Porn, rendered acceptable and even desirable, shameless bigotry too is transformed into a kink.

In her short story 'Coming Apart', Alice Walker describes a Black husband coming to terms with the reality of pornography.

He concludes that 'where white women are depicted in pornography as "objects", Black women are depicted as animals. Where white women are depicted as human bodies if not beings, Black women are depicted as shit.'[7] Walker's distinction between 'objects' and 'animals' is crucial in coming to terms with how racism infiltrates our way of thinking.[8] The animalistic depiction allows, necessarily, for a kind of dehumanisation, being easier to exploit, coerce, punish and control animals rather than people. Audre Lorde sheds light on pornography as devoid of humanity, as 'sensation without feeling'.[9]

MAINSTREAMING RACISM

The racism begins with race and ethnicity being defining categories within Big Porn, encouraging us to watch our porn and see performers through a racial lens. The algorithmic business model requires coding, of bodies, races and sexual behaviours, mostly labelling women and their bodies from a male, heterosexual point of view. Race, as with specific acts, is a selling point, commercialising the objectification of people based on their racial and ethnic backgrounds. A study of the most popular video tags on one of the largest mainstream platforms is one of the few studies that can tell us with some certainty about this process of rigid, racist categorisation.[10]

Of the 145 most popular tags, twenty-two referred to race or national identity, including Black girls, Indian girls/teen and Asian teen, with seven specifically referring to Japanese scenarios and actors. The only other national identities were Indian (two tags) and Thai (one). All the rest referred to broader categories such as African, Arab/Arabian, Asian, Muslim, Latina and Black, as well as interracial. A cursory visit to the most popular porn websites confirms this categorisation, such as XVideos, which offers up sixty-three main content categories, of which eight are based on race and nationality, a similar proportion to the study just discussed.

These labels show that there are overlaps between race, ethnicity and nationality. Common searches in any country tend to include nationality; many want to watch porn supposedly involving women from their communities and it doesn't make a difference to the nature of the pornography. However, sometimes it does, such as the dominance of Korean women being targeted in deepfake sexual abuse. It may be that 'Japanese' is being used as a proxy for particular types of pornography, such as hentai, stylised explicit anime in which highly sexualised imagery of young girls is common, or simulated child sexual abuse where women actors with small bodies are often in videos depicting underage-looking girls.

We must note here that the categories of race and ethnicity are minoritised from a Global North perspective. That is, it is predominantly the race and ethnicity of Black and brown women and men that is identified. There is hardly ever a reference to 'white'. Indeed, we tend only to see the label 'white' in a potentially racist context, such as the video viewed 17 million times on XVideos, entitled 'white cops fuck ebony teen'. The reality is that if you search for any particular sex act you will be presented first with white performers; to see Black and brown bodies, you need to search using racial labels. When Black and racially minoritised actors are in videos, this is almost always in the title. Whiteness is the default.

Another common label is 'interracial', and Pornhub's second most popular pay-per-view niche channel, boasting three million subscribers and 2.6 billion views, is Blacked.[11] However, in case you thought otherwise, Blacked is not a celebration of racial identity; this interracial material is not about sex between equals. This is something being done to white women by Black men depicted as hypersexualised, aggressive, dangerous: 'You, white woman, have been Blacked.'[12]

A particular form of this interracial material is 'cuckold', where men watch their partners have sex with other men. This can take many forms, but much of the interracial cuckolding takes on a sinister, 'rape-adjacent' projection with scenes typically containing multiple Black men and a single white woman.[13] It's important to understand that this material is primarily produced for white men (that's clear from the marketing, tags and commentary). It's a projection of racist views, corroborating their racial anxieties, seeing hypersexualised Black men having sex with 'their' white women. It's also misogynist and racist in its take on white women 'betraying their race'.[14]

These racist stereotypes of Black men's sexuality as aggressive, dangerous or animalistic are confirmed in a recent study finding that Black men were four times more likely to feature in an aggressive title than with white men, and they were three times more likely to appear in videos depicting visible male aggression.[15] This can be seen in videos described as involving blonde teens being 'ambushed' by a 'huge black man'. In addition, there's a particularly objectifying and derogatory way race is described in some material, including 'sexy blond teenage girl with loads of Blacks'. These and similar titles are all ways of insinuating 'force' or 'rape'. Simply identifying the man as

Black conjures up the threat of assault and rape; they don't need to say it explicitly.

The 'Big Black Cock' category is perhaps the most well-known; there are many references to 'monster black cock'. Black porn performers themselves try to challenge these stereotypes, encouraging us to understand the historical roots of the slave auction, when white people 'would try and choose men with the largest penis, because they felt they would breed the best'.[16] On XVideos, 26.8 million have watched 'teen annihilated by big black cock'. We see here the layers of racist power dynamics in operation: youth, force, racism, there for you to experience as part of a community of millions, all in the service of the profits of Big Porn.

There are also continued references in this content to the wider political context of racism, such as material referring to the Ku Klux Klan and eroticising police brutality in the US.[17] There's no getting away from such depictions having political connotations, and the influence can be seen through the eager and approving participation in the comment sections.

In terms of research, there is little on the specifics of race in pornography, particularly in the last few years, but what there is commonly focuses on aggression, such as findings that where videos depict Black men in sexual activity with white women, there are far higher levels of non-consensual storylines.[18] This reinforces age-old public attitudes associating Black men with violence and criminality, fulfilling the roles of criminals such as burglars and drug dealers, projecting damaging perspectives of Black culture being predominantly lawless, illegitimate and dangerous.[19] In the content study I undertook with colleagues, we found that the term 'Black' was more common in material depicting physical assault and coercion, suggesting another connection between sexual scripts of sexual assault and racialised descriptions of Black performers.[20]

Black women are variously presented as exotic, animalistic or not worthy of respect.[21] They are hypersexualised, as having an insatiable appetite for sex, particularly with white men.[22] In addition, young Black girls are 'adultified', meaning they are seen as less innocent, more sexual, legitimising a rougher approach with young-looking girls.[23] We also see racism, sexism and classism intersect, playing out in scenarios where the women are described using terms such as 'dumb', 'bitch' and 'from the ghetto'.

While Black women are often the targets of more acts of aggression than white women,[24] other research suggests similar levels of physical aggression towards Black and white women performers.[25] Interestingly, however, the authors of that study went on to reveal that Black women performers were the least likely group of women to experience *non-consensual* aggression.[26] Black women are portrayed as *wanting* aggression that no white woman would willingly undergo. White women are portrayed as helpless victims; Black women are portrayed as getting what they deserve and desire. You don't need me to tell you how dehumanising this is.

In contrast, women labelled 'Asian', sometimes categorised as 'oriental', are often referred to as submissive, passive, tiny, obedient, fetishised as 'exotic' objects of desire, reinforcing stereotypes about their roles in relationships and society. Content studies have found that Asian women are depicted differently from other women, often treated less aggressively and with far less agency, such as 'Asian fucktoy gets used in front of boyfriend'.[27] On the other hand, another study found that Latina and Asian women performers experienced higher rates of aggression compared with those involving white or Black women.[28] In most videos, Asian women were portrayed as passive, submissive or eager to please, perhaps the subject of more aggression because of these traits. Their lack of resistance is perceived as encouragement, and even when they do show discomfort or pain, this is likely to be ignored. This replicates a much earlier review of rape porn websites that also found an overrepresentation of Asian women[29] and ties into other stereotypes of Asian women as passive, doll-like bodies to be used for sex.[30]

Another genre of pornography I want to discuss is 'hijab' porn.[31] While the hijab is a religious, not racial, symbol, there remains, in many Western, predominantly white communities, a conflation of Muslim dress, identity, religion and race. This material is an example of different ways that racialisation works, here blending political, religious and racist stereotypes, forms of discrimination and violence. A recent porn content analysis found high levels of aggression towards Muslim women, and in almost all the videos, they were depicted as submissive, showing the inter-relationships between racism and patriarchy. They were predominantly portrayed as being exploited, reinforcing social stereotypes and scripts about Muslim immigrant women in Global North societies, such as the suggestion that these 'poor' women will do 'anything' in exchange for money, shelter and/or food.[32] In my content study, we similarly found examples of 'hijab' porn with a focus on exploitation, with titles such as 'Hijab wearing amateur lured into sex for cash'. Further, we know that participating in such porn can have serious consequences for the actors, as we saw in the case of Mia Khalifa, who was pressured into performing in a hijab, a video that has since defined and shaped her professional life.[33]

IMPACTS OF RACIALISED SEXUAL SCRIPTS

The overall picture is one of mainstream porn imbued with racism and racist stereotypes, with significant implications for Black and racialised women and girls. When investigating online misogynoir – the combination of racism and misogyny – the organisation Glitch reported that 'men indicate that they explicitly want to have sex with a Black woman, often because Black women are hypersexualised and therefore said to be more promiscuous'. They also found a lot of sexually explicit language online linking Black women to food such as 'chocolate'.[34]

Glitch reported that these attitudes and stereotypes are normalising the perpetration of sexual violence against Black women and girls, suggesting that they 'enjoy rape or provoke rape'.[35] The sexualised racism of porn, and its representation of Black women as welcoming violence, as well as their dehumanisation, may be putting Black women and girls at risk of significant harms. Their attempts to secure redress through criminal justice systems are often met with disbelief, lack of interest and discriminatory attitudes, in turn adversely impacting on the decisions of police, prosecutors, judges and juries. Sexual scripts of dehumanisation, hyper-sexualisation and higher levels of aggression against Black women and girls contribute to minimising and normalising such violence, sustaining a societal context devaluing Black women.

The impact of viewing racist porn has complicated impacts on Black women and girls' own sexual pleasure. The ways our sexual scripts are shaped by the world around us means that, for some, their sexual arousal is bound up in some of the same racialising structures and meanings that they otherwise reject.[36] Black women have talked about how seeing themselves and their bodies represented in porn, and as desirable, is a welcome celebration of Black women's sexuality, rather than being portrayed as second-class to other (white) women.[37] The Black Sexual Economies Collective talks about how Black sexualities are rendered 'both desirable and deviant' through their exploitation and appropriation in mainstream porn.[38] These perspectives complicate women's interactions with pornography and the messages it conveys.[39] But we must be mindful of how the rhetoric of individual choice has been co-opted by Big Porn, with *Playboy*'s founder Hugh Hefner once claiming to be at the forefront of ending racist stereotypes by 'portraying women of colour as sex objects to a predominantly white male readership'.[40]

For others though, searching for women that look like you in porn is more traumatic than arousing, as Black and racially minoritised bodies are so fetishised and hypersexualised.[41] One South Asian woman reports such experiences, with the racial categorisation of porn feeding the 'nasty racist stereotypes' we already have in society, leaving her feeling very uncomfortable. Her use of porn is reduced to finding the 'least offensive video possible'.[42] Not exactly the empowering, exciting, sex-positive smorgasbord of choice and empowerment that is sold to us.

FIGHTING RACISM IN THE PORN INDUSTRY

The blurring between on- and off-screen racism in porn has real effects on the porn industry. Writer and performer Zahra Stardust talks about how algorithmic tagging and ranking systems in mainstream porn 'benefit white performers and afford lower visibility and earning potential' to Black and racially minoritised performers, perpetuating a 'racial stratification' of the industry.[43] Not only are Black performers commonly paid less, but some non-Black women performers demand higher rates to work with Black actors, a premium known as an 'interracial rate'.[44]

There are performers who refuse to engage in the obviously racist material, only working with Black and minoritised actors when race is not the story or backdrop. However, the everyday reality makes this very difficult. Former porn actor Tyler Knight has talked about how, as a Black performer, he was continually trapped within rigid racial dynamics, with the vast majority of his work 'interracial'. Other Black actors have shared similar experiences, with Black porn performer King Noire saying the majority of his roles have been 'rooted in racism and colonialism'.[45] He emphasised that these racist tropes are not unique to porn and are reproduced in mainstream films, television shows and most popular media. Nonetheless, in porn, they are intensified in nature and impact, sexualising and eroticising what is otherwise commonly condemned or at least critiqued.

Some Black and racially minoritised porn performers are seeking to resist these portrayals, engaging in alternative interpretations, finding 'pleasure in Blackness'.[46] In 2020, many Black and minoritised porn performers came together to challenge the industry for its portrayal of racist tropes and use of racist terminology when labelling content, as well as the lower pay and status for Black performers.[47] In these ways, pornography with positive representations of Black and minoritised actors may have a role in destabilising narrow, stigmatising and otherwise oppressive standards of sexuality and pleasure. Therefore, just as porn creates and reproduces harmful sexual scripts, it might yet produce more egalitarian ones. However, as with indie and feminist porn discussed later in this book, while these are positive movements, they remain on the fringes, unfortunately making few indents into the vast swathes of racist, patriarchal porn.

Things are shifting a little, it seems. Mainstream articles reporting on race and pornography have headlines such as 'porn sites bolster racist tropes by design'.[48] Many working in the industry endorse this view. When discussing the spike in viewing 'cop porn' following the death of George Floyd and the #BlackLivesMatter protests, porn actor Jessa Jordan said it's 'dangerous, naïve and wildly privileged to choose to divorce the reality of police brutality from detention porn as entertainment'.[49] This was echoed by another performer who suggested that separating the two 'screams privilege and ultimately makes one complicit'. It's more than 'just entertainment'.[50] In the context of the importance of sex education, there's acceptance that this needs to include how porn disseminates damaging tropes about race that might be shaping people's understandings and expectations of Black and racially minoritised people.[51]

MAKING THE UNACCEPTABLE ACCEPTABLE

Porn fetishises racial differences. Being white is normalised, unseen, whereas race and ethnicity only has value in so far as it provides some variety and exoticism, a bit of difference to the 'standard' and 'boring' white female body. As the Black intellectual feminist writer bell hooks has said, 'Within commodity culture, ethnicity becomes spice, seasoning that can liven up the dull dish that is mainstream white culture.'[52] Mostly, the spice is increased levels of aggression and exploitation, and reproducing narratives around racism and inequality.

This has wider political implications, as racist porn is imbued with the culture of slavery, colonialism and discrimination, messages that inevitably seep into everyday interactions and attitudes, adversely impacting on our politics and economic futures. It was only a few years ago that Google's keyword library, which helps advertisers choose search terms to link with their adverts, associated searches relating to 'Black girls', 'Latina girls' and 'Asian girls' with porn.[53] Searches for 'white girls' did not have the same results. Built into Google's tech was a racial bias equating Black and minoritised women with sexualised representations. As well as demonstrating the stereotypical and discriminatory associations in AI and online between race and pornography, this has had broader economic and egalitarian impacts for girls and women. These biases make it more difficult for advertisers and companies to market their products to this group. Black and minoritised women are losing out in everyday life.[54]

This was not the first time Google had been called out for this sort of tech bias. Back in 2012, Safiya Noble demonstrated that searches for 'Black girls' regularly featured porn sites.[55] This again showed both the absence of data online about Black girls in all sorts of other contexts, as well as the close reproduction of hypersexual tropes around Black women and girls. While Google has fixed both of these problems, they are not alone. In fact, they are simply emblematic of the wider racism embedded in Big Tech and Big Porn, and becoming ever more evident in the roll-out of AI.

While the sexualised racism of decades ago was blatant and horrific, it was not being reproduced on the vast scale we now see in Big Porn. The ubiquity of porn, and of racial categories and stereotyping in mainstream porn, has taken this to new levels, reproducing these harmful narratives to millions every day. What once might have repelled us as racist is now resold to us as just another fetish or kink. However, what goes unquestioned in the realm of sex, relationships and attraction becomes harder to dismantle in other spheres of life. Big Porn is making the unacceptable acceptable.

5

Breathless

GRAHAM COUTTS HAD A TASTE FOR VERY SPECIFIC TYPES OF porn. He liked it when women were being strangled, with hands, tights or scarfs. He liked it when they stopped breathing, or at least looked like they had. He accessed this material through internet searches such as 'death by asphyxia' and 'sexy, strangled, suffocated, hanged'. Luckily for him, he had little difficulty finding this material online.

We know about this particular man's porn habits because, not long after searching for such material, he murdered a young woman, Jane Longhurst, by strangling her during sex with a pair of tights. He claimed it was an accident, the now familiar 'rough sex gone wrong' defence. The jury didn't believe him, though, and he was convicted of murder.

That was over twenty years ago, and when the details of his porn use were revealed at trial, it sent shock waves across society. Few knew that such material was easily and freely available on the internet. I didn't. We were only just getting used to Google, and accessing the internet was still a bit of an ordeal; there were no smartphones, and few had computers at home. Following a campaign by Jane's mum, a new law on extreme porn was adopted targeting the strangulation porn Coutts had been viewing. It was now an offence to possess 'extreme' porn that also included images of necrophilia and bestiality. The new law didn't include pornographic images of rape – but that's the story of another campaign I'll come to later on.

To discuss the law reform, I was interviewed on BBC Radio 4's *Woman's Hour*. My notes from the time, with a lot of underlining, remind me that this material was 'not mainstream' but extreme, and that was why we could justify criminalising it. Fast forward twenty years and strangulation porn barely raises an eyebrow. Now more commonly known as choking, it's a staple of rough porn. So ubiquitous is it across our culture that if you type it into a search engine, results aren't even pornographic. 'Choke me daddy' brings up Amazon selling T-shirts with this emblazoned across them, as well as songs by popular artists extolling the virtues of choking a woman during sex.

This shift – how the extreme has become mainstream – is a serious concern. For one, medical evidence is clear that sexual choking/strangulation is affecting women's memory functions and cognitive abilities; it's damaging their brains. And that's on top of the more immediate risks of losing consciousness, strokes, bloodshot eyes, sore throats, headaches, dizziness and bruising. Like getting punched in boxing, or having your head repeatedly smashed in rugby, regularly restricting the blood or oxygen to your brain has potentially long-term consequences. But unlike in sports, the harms are not well-known, and regulation is scarce.

Is this because it's particularly harming young women and as a group they rarely get a voice in public debate? Probably. Is it also because there's a vast industry of patriarchal porn shaping and sustaining the view that choking/strangulation in sex is normal and arousing? We rarely question the harms in the things we take for granted, and sex is no exception.

CHOKING OR STRANGULATION: WHAT ARE WE TALKING ABOUT?

It's not new that men engage in 'erotic asphyxiation', the masturbatory practice of strangling oneself. It's a recognised paraphilia and does sometimes lead to death. However, what we are talking about here is the increasingly common practice of choking/strangulation by sexual partners.

At some stage, strangulation during sex morphed into 'choking', and that's how it's now commonly described. However, strangulation is the technically correct term to describe external pressure applied to the neck to restrict breathing or blood flow. It can involve one or both hands, a limb or a ligature (belt, cord, scarf). 'Choking' is the precise term for internal blockages of the throat and air passages, such as when food gets trapped in your throat, or in the pornographic context, when a penis in the mouth blocks airways, making you cough or be sick.

However, in porn, across social media, and in everyday conversation, most people use the term 'choking' to refer to the sexual practice of hands around the neck, rather than the technically accurate 'strangulation'. There's something interesting going on in the particular language here. Like others, I can't help but think that using the term 'choking' somehow makes it seem less serious, less of a worry, than strangulation. This is even more evident if we think of the word used for someone who does this: a 'strangler'.

That's definitely a scary term we associate with horror films, and clearly focuses on the role of the aggressor. Even rarer are the terms 'suffocation' and 'asphyxiation', which happen to accurately describe these sexual activities. Some won't even use 'choking'; they'll use the innocuous-seeming euphemism 'breath play'.

Yet, at the same time as this neutralisation of harm is going on, we are hearing more about strangulation in domestic abuse. The extent and harm are increasingly being recognised, with many countries, including England and Wales, now introducing specific laws targeting non-fatal strangulation.[1] This is because, as well as the high risk of harm, it's commonly unlawful, whether in the domestic abuse or sexual context. You can't consent in law to what is called 'actual bodily harm'. The Crown Prosecution Service provides guidance that this means injuries such as damaged teeth or bones, extensive or severe bruising or loss of consciousness. It can include injuries inflicted willingly in sexual contexts, such as in some forms of sadomasochism. There are some exceptions granted in the public interest, like being able to consent to injuries sustained in sport. But there's no such exemption for sexual acts. Therefore, when choking/strangulation causes 'actual bodily harm', you can't lawfully consent, and the acts themselves are therefore unlawful. This means that if something does go wrong, and the injuries are serious, the strangler may commit a criminal offence, and consent would not be a defence.

Regarding terminology, I'm using both 'choking' and 'strangulation'. That's because 'choking' is the word many people know and understand, while strangulation is what it really is, and there's no mistaking its seriousness. If that term worries us, that's a good thing. But why is it so concerning?

SO WHAT?

Back in the 1940s, a seriously dodgy study was carried out on male prisoners and schizophrenia patients.[2] The aim was to find out how quickly they lost consciousness when strangled by an inflatable cuff around their neck. The answer is very quickly, within six or seven seconds. In another case of classic academic understatement, the study says that the human brain is 'remarkably sensitive' to loss of blood and oxygen. One of the researchers even tested the cuff around his own neck when he was on his own, and he very nearly died.[3] Though deeply unethical by today's standards, the researchers were trying to support the war effort by finding out more about how pilots lose consciousness when there's a loss of pressure in their aircraft. They were also aiming to learn more about the use of strangulation in treating schizophrenia (answer: no, funnily enough, strangulation does not cure schizophrenia).

So why is this relevant to us today? It's the only study we have showing the immediate effects on men of strangulation. As well as losing consciousness very quickly, it tells us that after about five or six seconds, the subject is no longer able to move their eyes to track a moving finger; their gaze becomes fixed. The experiment was designed so that the men could release the inflated cuff themselves, but in fact many found that before losing consciousness they froze, unable to use their fingers to release the pressure. So they were conscious, but they could not move or communicate. Transfer this into a sexual situation and we can see that blocking blood flow to the brain – choking/strangulation – can quickly lead to loss of consciousness, but before that, the person may be conscious, but unable to indicate any distress or lack of consent, or move their body. You can see that this would make it impossible to withdraw consent.

While loss of consciousness is not common, nearly one in five who have been choked/strangled have experienced some 'alteration of consciousness', i.e. dizziness, during sexual strangulation.[4] In another study, nearly one third reported negative consequences such as not being able to breathe, having a sore throat, becoming unconscious and/or having bloodshot eyes.[5] There are many other adverse effects, including changes to vision, paralysis and miscarriage. Perhaps not surprisingly, the more someone is choked/strangled, the greater the health risks. In addition, they are significantly more likely to report poorer mental health, and it quickly worsens for those who've been choked/strangled five or more times.

What is also emphasised in these studies is that the risks vary depending on other medical conditions, being worse if you have high blood pressure or high cholesterol. Significantly, these are not conditions likely to be known, particularly among younger people. So you may not even know if you are in a higher risk category. All of these concerns are why, even among some BDSM communities, this is not a common practice, as the risks of serious harm and even death are well-known.[6]

Nonetheless, people do report some positive experiences from suppressed breathing, including enhanced arousal.[7] However, desire and arousal (certainly for women) is as much psychological as physical, impacted by social expectations of sex and sexual double standards.[8] The pleasurable light-headedness, therefore, may not necessarily be a physical reaction as much as a general arousal response. I wonder whether the experience would remain positive if there was greater knowledge of the risk of serious harm.

Research so far has demonstrated very serious immediate risks, such as unconsciousness, strokes and death, and then a range of other adverse consequences including light-headedness, sore throats, inflamed eyes and headaches. But what is now being found is that frequent sexual choking/strangulation can have long-term adverse effects on cognitive functions, information processing and memory function.[9] It risks causing brain damage, and it is predominantly affecting younger women, right when their brains are still developing. These studies are based on MRIs, not a survey to be dismissed as 'sex-negative' or as a result of 'moral panic' (unless you don't care about brain damage in young women). It's vital to note that these adverse impacts – as with all the other harms discussed – are not specific to non-consensual acts. The damage is caused whether you consent or not.

HOW WELL-KNOWN ARE THE HARMS?

The general assumption amongst young people seems to be that choking/strangulation is 'probably' safe, though women are more sceptical and talk about fearing losing consciousness.[10] Many say they 'probably' know the signs of injury, though it turns out this does not match the reality of possible adverse consequences, probably because most young women say they've never sought information about techniques, risks or safety. They say they rely on their partners to know, and on the assumption that it's safe. Yet men similarly struggle to identify the risks.

While it would be all too easy to blame the men here (and there does need to be some personal responsibility), the media and internet is full of misinformation. When researchers looked into the most popular articles returned in searches for things like 'how to choke someone safely', they found many distortions. While many of the articles did refer to the risks of choking/strangulation, including death, they carried on talking about it as exciting, sexy and normal. For example, one key – inaccurate – message was that choking/strangulation is safe so long as done to the sides of the neck (rather than the trachea, the windpipe). However, this message that there are 'safe' ways to do it does not stand up to medical scrutiny.

The advice columns are also riddled with misogyny, with one of the most popular articles goading the reader: 'are you man enough to dominate her'. Another said, 'a lot of guys are afraid they're going to hurt a woman when they choke her ... but in reality that's part of the "danger" that women crave'. Researchers, steeped in knowledge of the real harms of choking/strangulation, were quite stark in their conclusions. The discussion of harms was alarmingly casual, with a 'sense that women's lives were not valued'. Doing it 'safely' seemed to imply just not killing the other person, which, as the authors say, is a 'shockingly low bar for sexual exploration'. As women are disproportionately the ones being choked/strangled, this 'amplifies the idea that women's lives are of less value than men's and speaks to a long legacy of misogynistic belief systems'.

CHOKING/STRANGULATION IN PORN: 'PLASTIC BAG BREATHPLAY EXTREME'

Once upon a time, there was very little choking/strangulation in mainstream porn. One of the earliest studies of porn content in the 1980s has no reference to it at all, despite an extensive list of aggressive acts being investigated.[11] It was just not a thing, certainly not apparent or worthy of study. Even the porn of twenty years ago, in the mid-2000s, had hardly any, with one study finding about 7 percent of material showing choking/strangulation.[12] However, by 2013–14, it was making its mark, being among the top five forms of physical aggression.[13]

Now, it's everywhere. As porn producer Erika Lust remarks, it's a standard way to have sex in mainstream porn.[14] In fact, it's so commonplace that it's difficult to determine exact statistics, as it's not always identified in titles, video tags or categories. For example, a Pornhub video titled 'I just want to please daddy' shows a man with two hands around the neck of a woman who looks to be in distress. This isn't labelled 'choking/strangulation', but that's what's shown to entice the viewer. It's difficult to determine exactly how common it is, because while 'choking' is the popular term generally used to describe strangulation, when used to label porn videos, the term is often describing choking on a penis. The porn websites use the medically correct term! Pornhub's algorithm is well aware of the confusion: type 'strangulation porn' into Google and it produces a Pornhub page headed 'Choke Strangulation Porn Videos' covering all angles.

One investigation into Pornhub's algorithm found that it presents more and more choking/strangulation porn to a new user, even when that's not what is being searched.[15] Pornhub's terms of service state that they do not remove content involving violent sexual acts, only 'extreme violence posing a serious risk of harm or death'. Yet a search for 'choke and porn' returns a Pornhub webpage labelled 'extreme choke porn videos'. Searches for 'strangle' are blocked on Pornhub, but not 'strangulation', and on one page headed 'choke me daddy' there are videos with strangulation involving belts tied around necks and videos labelled 'professor only lets me breathe when he thinks I deserve it'. There's a video where a plastic bag is tied tightly over the woman's face: 'More latex breathhood play'. What then do they consider 'extreme violence'?

As ever, X provides a remarkable amount of this material, with the misogyny and humiliation centre stage, and little pretence that it's pleasurable (for the woman). There are videos encouraging you to make the woman 'froth from the mouth', and if that's not happening, *you're not choking it hard enough*. The level of harm is obviously a concern, but the dehumanisation – choking *it* – is so stark.

WHAT'S THE INFLUENCE OF CHOKING/ STRANGULATION PORN?

Engaging in sexual choking/strangulation is far more common in people under thirty.[16] It's not difficult to think this might be due to its prevalence in Big Porn. Indeed, one recent study of over 4,000 Australians reported that porn was the primary source for learning about sexual strangulation.[17] In another survey, more than half of the men said pornography had influenced their desire to engage in rough sex including choking/strangulation, with one in five saying it had influenced them a 'great deal'.[18]

Another study looked into this more, finding that consuming pornography more frequently leads to greater exposure to pornographic depictions of sexual choking/strangulation, which, in turn, predicted a higher likelihood of strangling sexual partners.[19] So here we have a clear link between exposure to choking/strangulation in porn and undertaking the acts.

What is more, the sexual scripts pornography is producing are encouraging men to perform acts portrayed as pleasurable, safe and so normal that they don't require specific consent. This echoes the study I discussed earlier, where viewing rough sex in pornography is positively correlated with desire for, and engagement in, rough sex behaviours.[20] From the other side of the stranglehold, women report much the same, talking about how the first person who choked/strangled them was someone who watched it in pornography.

There are of course so many influences on our behaviour and sexual activity. As with rough sex, choking/strangulation is a cultural phenomenon, promoted and encouraged across social media and popular culture as exciting. However, while pornography and popular culture are closely intertwined, it is pornography where most people learn about sex. Big Porn is conveying messages about there being no need to seek specific consent: women will (eventually) like it, and it's safe.

WHO'S DOING IT AND WHAT'S THEIR REACTION?

It's perhaps, therefore, no surprise that choking/strangulation is far more common than it used to be, particularly among younger people. One study of US students found that around half had engaged in choking/strangulation, with a third of women reporting this during their most recent sexual activity. Just to emphasise, this study was just about their *most recent* activity, not sexual activity in general. Indeed, other research has found that 13 percent of sexually active girls aged 14–17 have already been choked/strangled. Figures from Australia show around half of those surveyed had been choked/strangled at some stage, with similar numbers strangling someone.[21]

The most recent data from the UK found that just over one third of young people have been choked/strangled during sex, a much higher proportion compared to those over thirty-five.[22] As well as it being commonplace, it's a gendered practice. More men choke/strangle their partners than do women, and choking/strangulation is experienced disproportionately by women, as well as sexual and gender minorities.

That's how common it is, but how is it experienced? When investigating rough sex in the UK, a BBC survey found that one in five women said they'd been left feeling frightened or upset after consensual rough sex experiences involving slapping, choking, gagging or spitting.[23] Emma shared her experience with the BBC, saying, 'we ended up in bed and during sex – without warning – he started choking me. I was really shocked and felt terrified. I didn't say anything at the time because at the back of my head, I felt vulnerable, like this man could overpower me.' In addition, the research found that nearly half of the women who experienced these forms of rough sex, during what they considered consensual sex, felt pressured, coerced or forced into it. This is telling us something serious, not only about how women are feeling during these sexual activities, but also that they are still describing this as consensual sex, even when being pressured, coerced or forced. I'm not doubting that they consider these to be consensual encounters. However, these results underline for me the inadequacy of consent as an arbiter of what is good, ethical, enjoyable sex.

This concern is confirmed in a US study finding that nearly one in four women said they felt scared during consensual sex, with choking/strangulation one of the most common causes of this fear, and with partners doing it without warning. It's unfortunately quite common for women to report being choked/strangled where their partner assumed consent.[24] In another BBC investigation, this time questioning 2,000 UK men aged 18–39, one third reported that they would not ask their partner for explicit consent prior to engaging in 'rough sex', including choking/strangulation.[25] This is echoed in a survey of 2,300 people, where only around half of those who have been choked/strangled said that consent was always discussed in advance.[26] This is deeply concerning, but we have to try to understand this in a context where these practices are normalised.

One woman, Laura, spoke to writer Rachel Thompson about when a man tried to choke/strangle her, without any discussion, on their first night together.[27] She said she 'just felt his hands around my throat all of a sudden'. Abigail similarly shared her experience of a man choking/strangling her; she didn't have the breath to be able to tell him to stop and she didn't want to make a fuss. She felt so confused and uncomfortable about the whole experience.

Rachel herself has talked movingly about her own experiences of being choked, of a man sitting on her chest, his penis in her mouth, when she feared for her life and could hardly breathe, but then not being able to understand or explain her feelings. 'Perhaps this is normal and I'm being weird,' she thought. She had a visceral fear that she might die, but she liked this man, had agreed to sexual activity with him, and so didn't share her experience with anyone else. Indeed, she told her friend that it was great sex. She was nineteen at the time, and didn't see her experience as anything out of the ordinary; she had no vocabulary to express it or explain it, yet fear defined many of her early sexual experiences.

Rachel speaks eloquently about the loneliness that comes from not being able to speak about these things, and that for so long she didn't realise that other women were silently trying to deal with the very same thing.

There's a confusing picture emerging here where the standard of consent really does not work for women. While some are saying they ask to be choked/strangled, finding some pleasure in it and therefore engaging voluntarily, others speak of not asking to be choked/strangled or seeking it out, but eventually coming to accept it, complying with the social cultural pressures.[28] Many talk about feeling uncomfortable, and the practices being unwanted, but they still consider it consensual. Understandably, they are not calling their experiences assault, with all the mental anguish that comes from such a label.

Even when there is consent, this is a very low bar, and doesn't engage with issues of want, joy or pleasure. Women talk about a standard of consent that includes 'assumed because normal', describing common experiences where the person choking/strangling simply presumed consent in the absence of any clear communication. The idea of consent, therefore, does not capture many women's experiences, where the sexual activity is not welcome or wanted. Is this the impact of patriarchal porn, where women's consent, and pleasure, is largely irrelevant, and they are shown as wanting and accepting almost anything?

PARALLEL UNIVERSES

We seem to be living in two parallel universes. The first is the world where choking/strangulation is common in young people's sexual lives, assumed to be safe, and normalised. Popular culture reinforces and reproduces these messages with supposedly humorous memes and hashtags, such as #chokemedaddy, as well as popular songs such as Jack Harlow's 'Lovin on Me', which refers to choking as vanilla, and has nearly 200 million views on YouTube. Many women speak of consenting, though this is as much about not labelling it as unlawful and some form of assault, rather than meaning the acts are wanted or enjoyed. There's a darker underbelly to this universe, of influencers in the manosphere normalising and encouraging this practice, characterising it as ultra-masculine, goading men into it, exemplified by notorious 'manfluencer' Andew Tate, who glorifies choking/strangulation.[29]

The other universe is the one where strangulation – as it is called here – is acknowledged as seriously harmful. First in relation to domestic abuse, the role of strangulation in the killing of women, as well as a means of abuse and control, is increasingly being recognised worldwide through the introduction of new laws targeting non-fatal strangulation. Strangulation in this context is recognised as a significant predictor of homicide. Sentencing guidelines start from the position of the 'inherent harm' of strangulation.[30] Then, in the law enforcement context, not least following the death of George Floyd sparking #BlackLivesMatter, the chokehold or stranglehold is commonly now banned, as it's so risky.

We need to bring these worlds together. The medical message of there being no safe way to strangle someone needs more prominence. One research project with students did find that, while they at first thought choking/strangulation was safe, after discussion of the medical evidence revealing the harms, the positive perceptions were reduced.[31] Not surprisingly, it was women who particularly took on board these messages, because, of course, they are mostly the ones being strangled. There's a real appetite for more information and discussion about choking/strangulation, as I found out when I posted a video on TikTok talking about sexual strangulation giving young women brain damage. It went viral, being viewed 1.4 million times (the vast majority being women under thirty-five), with thousands of comments and likes. Nearly forty thousand shared the video, showing a real desire to share this information and discuss what is happening, with many commenting that they'd had no idea this was so risky, and they'd thought at first my video was a humorous meme.

Men also need to challenge themselves and their peers more. They need to ask themselves why they want to run the risk of causing irreversible harm or even death for sexual gratification. They need to understand that obtaining consent does not absolve them of their ethical, and indeed legal, obligations to other human beings. Quite frankly, this is in their own best interests, unless they want to face a knock on the door from the police down the line.

BUT WHAT ABOUT CONSENT?

When you talk openly about the risks of choking/strangulation, people will be quick to accuse you of stigmatising the sexual choices of consenting adults. If women choose to be choked/strangled, it's claimed, who are you or the law to step in and say they can't enjoy themselves? I've discussed how the contractual language of consent doesn't suffice when it plays out in a cultural context where women feel they have few meaningful alternatives. That is, a cultural context where many prospective male sexual partners expect to be able to choke/strangle them. And women are typically reluctant to describe sexual encounters that they initially consented to as assault. Yet they feel harmed, disturbed and a deep sense of unease. Some feel scared during sexual activity, fearing the worst. They convince themselves that this is what is expected; this is what social media and porn is saying, and so they come to accept it. Women might not find pleasure in sexual activity, but they comply.

Some will object to me describing things this way, emphasising their genuine willingness. But attempts to draw a clear line between consensual and non-consensual choking/strangulation doesn't settle questions of some women's uncomfortable state of mind. While some of the disturbing experiences are due to the lack of consent, many others are not understood as assault, but they are still deeply unnerving. This is why young women are increasingly discussing the pressures they feel.[32] Simply making the seeking and giving of consent clearer won't make those feelings go away. These emotions are present because choking/strangling is not a neutral action – it is inherently an act of dominance; it's a threat to someone's life. It doesn't feel right because many women can sense that, when they are being choked/strangled, it's not about their pleasure or what they want. Instead their partner is exercising power over them, consensually or not. You can agree to being at someone's mercy, but it doesn't make you any less vulnerable.

The patriarchal air we breathe cloaks this sense of unease. The dominance of 'consent culture' denies any space for ambivalence.[33] The allure of what's labelled sex-positive, being wanted, being cool is being driven home by mainstream porn playing it well, making women doubt themselves, and convincing them that this is in fact sexy, wanted, normal, safe.

Then there's the dimension of harm. Even if clearer consent magicked away the sense of unease, the reality of the physical harms of choking/strangulation remains. Maybe this is why you're getting more headaches, why it seems you're finding it harder to concentrate than you used to? It's got immediate risks, as well as potentially significant long-term effects, the full extent of which we don't yet know. Young women are the unwitting guinea pigs in a mass experiment. And the misinformation paraded across the internet should make us concerned about how little women's lives and well-being are valued. Finally, even if someone consents, during the acts they may well be unable to withdraw consent as their body goes into shock, unable to respond or show concern. Safe words don't help you if you can't speak.

FROM SIMONE DE BEAUVOIR TO BARBIE

Living in a patriarchal world can be confusing and bewildering. Think of the famous speech in the *Barbie* film where Gloria, played by America Ferrera, talks about the impossible double standards of being a woman, of being so tired of watching yourself and every other woman tie themselves in knots so that people will like them, want them, so that they can fit in, be accepted. To be sexy but not too sexy, to want sex but not too much or with too many people. To relish danger but not actually want to be killed or suffer brain damage.

Laying the groundwork for *Barbie*, seventy or so years earlier, French philosopher Simone de Beauvoir talked of life for women under patriarchy being one of 'inner uncertainty and confusion'.[34] Women are trying to live with the shock and ambiguity about what is really happening to them, being just so different from what they are being told is happening to them. We're being told by society and porn that behaviours such as choking/strangulation, and other forms of rough sex that privilege men's sexual desires and satisfaction is all normal and what we should want. Yet this doesn't reflect how many feel.

With choking/strangulation, it's almost like women are being given a slow-acting drug to incapacitate them, hoping they won't notice. It's a ticking time bomb. As a practice, it is literally holding women in their place, damaging brains, limiting physical and mental resistance to the world we live in, all the while convincing women it's what they want. That's the strength of patriarchy: gendered inequality thrives through its eroticisation, making women think it's sexy.

6

Barely Legal

THERE WERE TIMES WHEN WRITING THIS BOOK THAT I THOUGHT I might not be able to carry on. One of those times was finding the video on Pornhub entitled '4-foot-6 rough fuck makes tiny TikTok teen squirt'. From the image of the very young-looking girl, and the use of the word tiny, I guessed the intention. But I had to look up the significance of '4-foot-6'. Turns out this is the average height of a ten-year-old girl. Here was a video, in plain sight on Pornhub, advertising itself as featuring someone looking like a ten-year-old girl. This video had been viewed 10 million times. You can type '4-foot-6 porn' into Google, Pornhub, XVideos and others, and they provide you with many pages of this type of material.

Finding this whole genre of '4-foot-6' porn derailed me at first. Feeling powerless in the face of its ubiquity and popularity, I posted about it on X in an attempt to at least raise awareness. Responses included the suggestion I had made it up (they clearly haven't heard of Google or gone on X, where you can also find this video), and more commonly that it didn't matter, as the actors would be over eighteen and this is 'fantasy'. The young woman in this particular film is in fact a well-known porn actor. Perhaps this was why so many had already watched the video? But does that make a difference? Many watching it will know this is someone over eighteen, yet I remain troubled by this being promoted as a very young-looking girl, and a very young girl being 'rough fucked'. Many others will not know this is a well-known actor and may view the material because it is popular and highly ranked, and algorithmically suggested to them; or they may have sought it out as their preference is for depictions of young girls.

This chapter is about the category of 'teen' in Big Porn, sometimes known as 'barely legal', and what this tells us about the porn industry, about users, about the effects on girls and society generally. While Big Porn tries to justify the label 'teen' as being about eighteen- and nineteen-year-olds, we all know this is not the whole story. While we might like to draw a bright line between child sexual abuse material (bad and criminal) and legitimate adult porn (good or at least OK and lawful), this is not possible. There is a murky, disturbing overlap, where viewing teen and barely legal material does and should give you the unsettling sense that all is not right, and that some of this material may well be unlawful.

WHAT'S OUT THERE?

First, we need to face up to the reality that child sexual abuse material is on the mainstream porn sites. *The Sunday Times* did a powerful exposé in 2019 showing how easily discoverable some of this material was on Pornhub.[1] We know it's available from the multiple lawsuits being taken against companies such as Pornhub by women whose images of childhood sexual abuse were uploaded and circulated online for many years before being taken down.[2]

While removal processes have improved, not enough has changed. A study in 2024 found that child sexual abuse material remains 'shockingly accessible' on the open web, particularly on Big Porn and social media.[3] Of those searching for child sexual abuse material, one third say they found this material on pornography websites, rather than the dark web, with Pornhub being the most common.[4]

As well as those deliberately looking for this material, a recent study found that almost one third of porn users have unintentionally come across sexual material involving children.[5] It's really not difficult to find. In just three clicks, investigators at the UK's National Crime Agency found abuse material via common search engines, showing that there are no barriers to offending on the open web.[6] Another investigation revealed pathways on TikTok and Instagram for those seeking this out.[7] Likewise, OnlyFans has come under scrutiny for hosting child sexual abuse material.[8]

It's vital therefore that we all understand that child sexual abuse material is relatively straightforward to find, as well as being easy to stumble across. But the next point is almost more important. This material is so easily findable because there is such an overlap between a much larger array of ostensibly lawful imagery – teen porn – and child sexual abuse material.

Teen porn often includes videos of very young-looking teenage or younger girls. These videos mimic child sexual abuse material, and some of it may well be. These are the images that stop you in your tracks and make you feel sick, worried that this is child sexual abuse material, wondering why are we allowing this promotion of sexual activity with young girls. The sorts of videos I'm talking about can be found across the most popular sites, from searches and suggestions relating to 'tiny', 'young' and terms such as '4-foot-6'. These terms produce videos referring to 'tiny sluts' who are 'abused', as well as 'schoolgirls' paying their debts with sex. Titles often also contain words indicating youth, such as 'pigtails', 'homework' and 'braces'. I am aware that some women over eighteen have braces, but let's be honest about why such words are used.

In case you are thinking – hoping – that this material is not common, the teen genre is one of the most popular on Big Porn. In my research, we trawled the landing pages of the three most popular porn sites, analysing 150,000 video titles, and found that, of all the words used, 'teen' was the most common across the entire dataset.[9] This means it was more common than the label for any sex act or body part. Other common words indicated youth, such as 'girl' and 'schoolgirl'.

We also know this is a common category from a recent study examining the most popular video tags on one of the most frequented porn websites. The most common 145 tags were used over 27 million times.[10] They included 'teen anal', 'chubby teen', 'old and young', 'petite' (a common euphemism for young girls), 'virgin', 'young girl', many labels for race and ethnicity, such as 'Asian teen', 'black girls', 'Indian teen', 'Japanese teen', and many incest and stepfamily labels, including 'daughter' and 'stepdaughter'. Tags specifically focused on being under-age and related to incest received 5.65 million hits. I share all of these tags just to convey the nature and range of themes relating to young girls that are so popular.

While steps have been taken on most mainstream sites to limit the most obvious searches for child abuse material, the efforts are largely performative. Type 'young girl' into Pornhub and you are blocked, but try 'girl young' are you are fine. Type 'very young' into Pornhub and you get a warning message. But try 'young' and you're fine. You then get offered 'tiny', then 'extra small', and so it goes on. You don't need a nuanced understanding of algorithms to work out that the sites take you to ever more extreme material, including simulated or authentic child sexual abuse imagery.

Teen porn therefore is a vast category of material in mainstream porn. Crucially, while some of it is about differentiating these videos from the category MILF (involving older women), it's far more sinister. There's a strong association between teen porn, sexual violence and aggression. In my research, we found that the word 'teen' is more common in sexually violent content, with titles referring to teens being 'abused' and made to cry.

While I've already talked about how much of mainstream porn is aggressive and violent, it's important to understand that this is even more so in teen porn. The actors are even more likely to experience degrading treatment and engage in risky sex acts, and are five times more likely to appear in forceful anal penetration scenes.[11] In addition, 90 percent of the teenage girls in videos containing visible aggression displayed pleasure, portraying these acts as both wanted and enjoyed.[12]

The term 'barely legal' unsurprisingly is not as common as it once was, perhaps because there's no plausible deniability about what it means. It used to be a much more accepted part of the mainstream porn industry, with the porn empire *Hustler* launching the bestselling magazine *Barely Legal* in the 1970s. But it remains available online, marketed via X and other social media, and its website claims it offers an 'exhilarating blend of innocence and allure' and the 'vibrancy of youth and the fire of first experiences'. Much of the material is based on the idea of 'first time'; babysitters are common, and age and power gaps are staples.

However, the barely legal material of a few decades ago differs from today's porn.[13] It was less violent and aggressive, the script being about grooming young girls into sexual activity (commonly with much older men), and therefore involved more 'intimacy', such as kissing, more encouragement and coaxing. One of the founders of *Barely Legal* talked about how the videos 'didn't need to be hard core and we were not competing with porn, this was some little innocent newbie playing with herself for the "first time"'.[14] There are many storylines involving 'defloration', innocence and loss of virginity and vaginal bleeding as evidence. These narratives of course pose serious threats to young women's safety and well-being too. But the teen material on Big Porn is commonly more violent, aggressive and body punishing. It's become more extreme, not just idealising sexual activity with young teenagers but glorifying sexually violent activity.

While the label 'barely legal' is no longer as common, it is seeing something of a revival in the promotion of AI girlfriends.[15] On X, #barelylegal brings up violent rape porn, with titles referring to 'force' and the woman saying no 'over and over'. There's far less moderation of titles on this site, with some referring to 'tiny girl'. This content is commonly tagged #agegap #virgin #forced and similar. Finally, as well as social media making teen and barely legal porn so accessible and seemingly legitimate, we must not forget about Google, which swiftly returns lots of this material and links to websites such as *tamedteens* and *dominateteens*.

NOT 'JUST' A FANTASY

There is no doubt that child sexual abuse material is openly trafficked on some of the more popular porn websites and across social media such as Instagram.[16] The opportunities to view this content are plentiful and require minimal effort from users of any age. No one needs to go to dedicated child sexual abuse sites, nor do they need knowledge of the dark web. This content doesn't have flashing lights and red alerts saying danger, danger, this is child sexual abuse content. It's just there, next to rough teen porn, young schoolgirl anal or whatever other teen porn is being watched. You can start on the category 'teen' and you're a few clicks away from both the lawful younger-looking and more violent material, *and* child sexual abuse content; though telling them apart is well-nigh impossible. Much as we may not want to admit it, the reality is that mainstream porn, particularly teen porn, is a pathway to viewing and accessing child sexual abuse material and other offending against children.[17]

Not only does this reality need to be recognised, we also need to understand how this happens. There's no dramatic crossing the Rubicon moment when a man stops watching 'ordinary' porn and becomes a paedophile watching child sexual abuse material. Researchers have concluded that the most striking characteristic of men who view sexual images of children is their 'ordinariness'.[18] The route is through incremental steps. Any single progression along the spectrum towards child sexual abuse content may not present a psychological threshold, or moral challenge, because it seems so easy.

This is not to suggest any lack of responsibility or agency of the individuals involved who are fuelling this trade. But it is to bring us back to the business model of Big Porn and the tenacious algorithms driving us to engage with more extreme content. In the context of child sexual abuse material, this is why people who didn't start out searching for child sexual abuse content find themselves doing so.[19]

Many studies of those who access child sexual abuse material have described how they initially start with watching mainstream pornography, progressing through pop-up adverts, repeated exposure, and then through to more extreme material, including child sexual abuse content.[20] These self-reports align with research on desensitisation, i.e. over time viewers become less sexually stimulated by mainstream sexual themes and seek out novel material.[21] Another study of users of child sexual abuse imagery found that 20 percent said that desensitisation to adult pornography was one reason they viewed this content.[22] In terms of teen porn, the Lucy Faithfull Foundation, which works with offenders to reduce child sexual abuse, is clear that viewing teen porn is leading to accessing and using child sexual abuse material and other offending against children. It's obvious really, we all know we build up a tolerance towards situations and media content the more we see it and get used to it, whether it's stories of war, famine, deaths or porn.

These pathways and the everyday nature of the (mostly) men accessing this material explain why the statistics are just so high. In 2021, the US National Center for Missing and Exploited Children, which removes this material from the internet, received nearly 30 million reports of child sexual abuse content.[23] However, the concern is that porn is not only a pathway to accessing child sexual abuse material but also to contact sexual offending. After viewing child sexual abuse content on the dark web, 40 percent of users said they had sought contact with a child, mainly using social media, gaming and messaging apps.[24] Another report examined risk factors of men who had sexual feelings for children or who had offended against children, and found they were eleven times more likely to watch violent pornography and twenty-seven times more likely to watch bestiality.[25] Another way of looking at this is that 22 percent of men who watched porn daily had sexually offended against children.[26]

There is also a strong correlation between accessing child sexual abuse content and engaging with other radical and extremist content online.[27] This reminds us of the connections between Big Porn and some of the misogynistic male influencer content that is being algorithmically pushed to younger men. We are seeing here the combined forces of the algorithmic drive to keep engagement through new, exciting, different, more extreme content, with the reality that we all become desensitised to what we are used to, and so look for something fresh.

As well as teen porn being a pathway to child sexual abuse content and offending, there is also the adverse impact on teenagers themselves, particularly young women. Girls have shared their reflections on the abundance of teen porn, with one describing how the 'schoolgirl trope in porn led me to being sexually harassed often', and another saying 'you see a lot of like barely legal teens on porn sites and it's not nice; they want us to act like porn models'.[28] This is particularly significant when Big Porn is such a common source of sex education and teen porn is even more aggressive (against the women and girls) than other genres. This means that young women are seeing aggressive and degrading acts associated with sexual pleasure, and indeed, as the norm for their age group. They may then feel pressure to enjoy (or at least pretend to enjoy) such acts. Young men may find such scripts limiting, as they seem to demand that they act aggressively if they wish to satisfy their partners' sexual desires.

It seems quite likely, therefore, that in sexual activities involving young people, both women and men are operating under the delusions inculcated by porn. This needs to be considered alongside the global statistics that sexual assault is committed against teenage girls more often than any other demographic group, with a significant spike between ages fourteen and seventeen.[29] In the UK, police receive more reports of rape from fourteen-year-old girls than any other age group. There is in fact a growing concern across many countries that are seeing increases in teenage boys sexually assaulting teenage girls, with porn being pinpointed as one explanation for why the statistics are getting worse.[30]

Finally, as with all forms of patriarchal porn, the ramifications go beyond harm to specific individuals and need to be understood at a societal level. The porn mimicking child sexual abuse material sends the message that it's legitimate to gain sexual arousal from children and child-like bodies and to sexualise them. The eroticisation of young teenage girls risks child sexual abuse not being taken seriously, with impacts and effects on related legal, policy and economic matters. What financial resources do we give police to focus on rape and child abuse? What about funds for local authorities dealing with abuse? How do we hold social media companies to account (if at all) for facilitating the creation and distribution of child sexual abuse material? How do police, judges and juries interpret and understand aggressive sexual activity between teenagers when it mimics a porn script? Answers to these questions are shaped by our environment, which includes the prevalence of teen porn and the messages it conveys. Is this contributing to the lack of attention to child sexual abuse? Is it why we are seeing more problematic sexual behaviour among teenage boys? Is it impacting on how victims understand their abuse and the (lack of) support they receive from their families and communities?

WHAT ABOUT REGULATION AND PREVENTION?

There is a lot to say about what needs to be done to better regulate the porn industry, as well as strengthening the criminal and civil law. But for now, I want to mention some specific projects that are underway to try to divert and help those who may be seeking child sexual abuse content.

Let's start with the actions of some of the platforms to block certain search terms that might indicate an interest in young children. As I've already mentioned, Pornhub and others do block some terms, but the effort is half-hearted. If we take Pornhub, its apparent interest in trust and safety is relatively recent. In documents released in one of the many lawsuits it's currently facing, we learn that one video uploaded in 2016, and only removed in April 2021, was classified by Pornhub moderators as involving prepubescent sexual acts and was tagged 'young', 'virgin-defloration' and 'teen'.[31] There are many other examples of material involving similar levels of extremity that were on the site for years, despite having been flagged for removal many times. An email between Pornhub employees in November 2020 stated that there is a 'LOT of very, very obvious and disturbing CSAM [child sexual abuse material] here', with another discussing in 2019 how the site permitted searches for 'very young teen', and that terms 'childhood' and 'minor' were to continue being allowed.[32] Top executives debated whether to ban 'little young girl' and 'very very young fuck'.[33] Yes, this was a *debate*, not just obvious.

Now, you may recall that in December 2020 Pornhub removed millions of videos after the furore following the *New York Times* article revealing the extent of unlawful material on the site.[34] Since then, it has prohibited many of the most obvious search terms.

Note, however, that some of this material remained online after December 2020. The Pornhub management remains much the same today as from before 2020.[35] While some of the more obvious terms are banned, many others are not, and even when a word is banned from a search, it is still permitted in titles and used in tags to facilitate the algorithm and further searches. Finally, while some of these English-language terms may be restricted, not so with many Spanish equivalents, including phrases referring to '13-year-old girls having sex'.[36]

Nonetheless, Pornhub have been involved in a positive collaboration with the Lucy Faithfull Foundation and the Internet Watch Foundation to use pop-up warnings and a chatbot to disrupt users who may be searching for child sexual abuse material. When UK users enter specific search terms, they are presented with a pop-up warning and given the opportunity to engage with a chatbot directing them to support services. A trial found that, when presented with the warning, some people did seek professional help.[37] It further revealed the scale of the issue. Over a period of eighteen months in the UK, the warning message was displayed 2.8 million times.[38] From the 2.8 million warnings, approximately 500 users transferred to the Lucy Faithfull's Stop It Now website. This might seem like there are millions who did not seek support. However, others who received the warning did carry on searching on Pornhub, but just for different imagery. It's also possible others will have read the message and perhaps changed their behaviour without seeking help.

This sort of initiative is significant, and we should all want it to succeed. It is good that Pornhub are working with others in this way, and that some users are getting help. It is, though, seriously concerning that some of the most common terms searched for included 'kids' or 'kid', 'young teen', 'child' or 'children', 'young girl', 'young boy', 'ddlg' ('daddy daughter little girl'), 'loli', 'little girl', 'Lolita' and 'child porn'.[39] These search terms reveal that people were unambiguously looking for sexually explicit material involving children.

There are other examples of how warnings may help divert users. A group of researchers created a men's health website, and when a user clicked on an advert for a 'barely legal' porn site, they got a warning message.[40] When the message implied the user needed help, such as 'concerned about your porn use?', the click-through to the barely legal porn website was significantly reduced. Overall, approximately half of those faced with the messages decided not to carry on to the barely legal website. While based on small numbers, this does point towards a relatively straightforward way to nudge users away from this material. A similar project found that deterrent messaging – that an IP address can be traced – was comparably effective.[41]

I highlight these projects as they point us towards actions that can be taken to try to divert those seeking child sexual abuse content, though sadly revealing the sheer extent of the problem. These projects should continue, and they should be further developed and supported. However, at the same time, I insist we do not get swept away by the positive PR. At the same time that Pornhub is participating in this project, the top-ranked search on Google for '4-foot-6 porn' returns Pornhub. Just for balance, the same search returns XHamster advertising 'tiny teen 4 foot 6 gets big cock' and XVideos offering 'tiny step daughter'. XVideos lists one of its tags that you can use to label videos or search for content as 'tiny girl'. Why do we put up with this?

WHY I HAD TO CARRY ON

I am not trying to be sensationalist or alarmist when I discuss this material, however uncomfortable it may be to read. I will even grant that teen porn, as a category, can include material that is not unduly problematic. Some of it just uses the 'teen' label to lure people in, and the content is little different from much other porn. However, lots of teen porn is deeply troubling. Some of it is authentic child sexual abuse material, though much of that is now removed when flagged. Yet it remains difficult to determine how much is out there when there is so much content mimicking child sexual abuse with very young-looking actors. While it may be declared fantasy by some, this content is normalising sexual activity with children. Its appeal is precisely in its resemblance to illegal and immoral sexual activity. Any such fantasy needs to be challenged, and help offered to change, not lauded, applauded and monetised by Big Porn.

Other teen porn plays on abusive sexual scripts commonly involving an age gap, and often involving exploitative relationships and incest. This is patriarchal porn living up to its label, eroticising the exercise of power by men over young, often vulnerable, women. This material risks leading men (and it is predominantly men) from ostensibly lawful teen porn towards unlawful content and possibly then to contact sexual abuse. It is also producing sexual scripts that teenage girls welcome aggression and violence, and that this is what is expected of teenage boys. Over time and with repetition, it dulls our sense of right and wrong. Porn viewers no longer see the boundaries they are crossing as they are drawn to more and more extreme material.

This is all very bleak, and I'm afraid that I am not able to lighten the load. Nonetheless, I started this chapter recounting one of many days when I thought I couldn't carry on writing this book due to the horrors of what I was viewing, and I'm going to end it with a story about one of the days when I knew I just had to carry on.

It starts on XVideos, one of the most popular porn sites across the world, and a search for 'teen', which brought up a video titled 'scared crying teen gets pounded'. This video involves sexual activity between a man and young woman bound with duct tape around her mouth and wrists; she's slapped, spat on, strangled at various times with two hands, as well as her nostrils being held closed while a penis is gagging her. This film is marketed as non-consensual – the title tells us she's scared and crying – and involves seriously dangerous acts, including strangulation and restricting her ability to breathe.

But it's the overall sense that is hard to convey here. This is not pink fluffy handcuffs from Ann Summers, but duct tape, reminiscent of kidnaps, trafficking and stranger rape. Crucially, the harm is not simulated; he's actually holding her nostrils closed while gagging her and he also uses *both* hands to choke/strangle her. While he has an erection, this has the feel of punishment, anger, resentment, loathing. Those are motivations for rape and sexual assault (it's not all about sexual gratification), so not surprising to me in some ways, but that's not what porn is supposedly about. This video has been viewed over 5 million times, has many supportive comments and is tagged 'punish', 'obey', 'helpless', 'rough', 'young'.

I watched this video on the same day that a man working for Ofcom, the body that regulates the porn industry, posted a job advert commenting that it would be of interest to someone who 'has always wanted to work in porn but doesn't have the feet for Only Fans'. I saw this and my jaw dropped. Here was someone in charge of regulating the sort of material I had just been viewing making a joke about working in the porn industry. Then it got worse when I realised that over thirty other Ofcom staff had liked the post, including some senior managers.

My outrage was shared by others and picked up by the media, resulting in an Ofcom apology (one mistake, of course we take our role seriously). I got my chance in the *Telegraph* newspaper and on BBC news to explain that, while I rail against the content on the mainstream porn sites, this almost felt worse, a gut punch.[42] It pointed towards a regulator and culture that had no real interest in, or commitment to, change, one that seemed not to understand the harmful nature of so much of the content on these platforms and the scale of the task ahead.

Granted, in terms of scandals and outrages, this is not that big. And while that individual felt entitled to make a joke online about working 'in' the industry, there are over 5 million people who have watched 'scared crying teen gets pounded'. It wasn't XVideos in the news being asked why this video is acceptable, or broader questions about the world we live in where over millions have watched it. The porn platforms are under the radar peddling this content with their avaricious algorithms, and hardly anyone is noticing or questioning it.

It was the juxtaposition of these two events that has driven me on. As well as the vital work raising awareness of the content of patriarchal porn, we must educate and motivate those who are supposed to be regulating the industry. Regulators are largely faceless, their existence and role hardly known to anyone. But I know who they are and what they should be doing; that's my job. So I needed to carry on. It's the regulator who sits between us and Big Porn, who has the power to challenge them, to hold them to account, to get them to remove – at the very least – all the unlawful and non-consensual material so easily and freely accessible.

I have kept going for the sake of all the 'scared crying teen girls' getting pounded, for the young men and boys being algorithmically fed the script that this is normal, and for the rest of us currently living with the normalisation of this violent eroticisation of young women. The stakes are too high to log off and just hope things might improve.

7

Family Ties

SEXUAL ABUSE BY FATHERS, STEPFATHERS AND (STEP)BROTHERS of young girls is among the easiest form of abuse to perpetrate, the hardest to uncover, and devasting for victims. It's a form of abuse that we rarely talk about. If we do talk about it, we are much happier discussing institutional abuse in religious communities, residential schools, sports coaching or care homes, or about well-known, celebrity serial abusers. Few want to be confronted with the reality that girls are at the highest risk of sexual abuse in the family home. It's the institution of the family that is most implicated in the sexual abuse of girls.[1]

Yet we watch porn reproducing this abuse in our millions. Forty years ago, there was hardly any incest in pornography. It's now one of the most popular genres. To hide from the reality, we give it names like 'fauxcest'. We search for it in categories like 'fosterfuck' or 'fucked up families'. We can see that videos referring to 'virgin stepdaughters' have over 7 million views, together with videos of very young-looking girls with dummies in their mouths and videos labelled 'teeny tiny' stepdaughter. On X, type in 'incest', and you get incest porn. No surprise that if you search for 'incest porn' on Google, you get pages of websites dedicated to this material.

In juxtaposing these two realities – the hidden harms of intra-familial sexual abuse of young girls and rampant levels of incest porn – I will be said to misunderstand the nature of sexual fantasy. Castigated for taking it all too seriously when it's so clearly not real. I'm well aware that (most of) these are videos with actors, some feeling squeamish about it, but recognising this is where the money is.

Nonetheless, I'm not prepared to accept this material as pure fantasy. The proliferation of incest porn is both a cause and a consequence of our societal apathy towards child sexual abuse. The pornification of incest, the frequency and casualness with which incest is portrayed in porn, normalises and minimises incest amongst viewers and society generally. It encourages us to supress our concern that this is wrong and harmful (those girls seem to like it). We take the reality of abuse less seriously, making light of victims' experiences.

As if that is not enough, incest porn reinforces the justifications and denials of abusers. If abusers were looking for some free propaganda that would help them deny the harm and shift responsibility, they couldn't have asked for more than an internet awash with incest porn. It gives credence to their claims of girls initiating sexual activity, of girls wanting to have sex with family members, of them enjoying it, of them not being harmed. In turn, these messages and norms influence us all, our choices, and decisions, just as it does those of law enforcement, of family support services, of juries, of journalists, of politicians and the media. The prevalence, and easy and free availability, of incest porn contributes to a society that does not take child sexual abuse seriously, does not object when governments take little interest in it or fail to invest in services working with victims and families.

UNDERSTANDING INCEST

I'm afraid I'm going to start this chapter by trying to understand incest a bit more. Bear with me: I get that you may have wanted to skip this chapter and that it may be very challenging for those who have experienced this form of abuse. But we must confront this, to understand why there is so much incest porn online now and what we can then do about it. We mustn't keep turning a blind eye, giving up because it is just so common or because we just can't face it.

Despite incest being prohibited in most societies, significant numbers of women and young girls are still victims of this abuse. To understand why, we can go back to Freud dismissing the accounts of women, suggesting the high incidence of father-daughter incest being reported was 'hardly credible'.[2] He simply did not want to believe it and so he didn't. He told everyone else the same and his followers continued to explain disclosures of abuse as girls fantasising about sexual activity with their fathers. Incest was hidden, denied, ignored.

When it was not possible to dismiss all the reports as fantasy, then ideas of complicity and blame took over. In the 1940s, influential research talked about how survivors did not deserve the 'cloak of innocence', with young girls being said to assume an 'active role in initiating the relationship', and that the girl victims were often 'unusually charming and attractive in their outward personalities'.[3] This 'participation' was then used to suggest that there were few long-term negative effects on children.

As well as the girls being willing, incest was justified by mothers withholding sex from their partners, meaning the father has to, is entitled to, seek sexual services elsewhere within the family. So the girls are asking for it and the wives are denying it. It's clear the men have no choice… One study declared that the wives of incestuous fathers were 'not only frigid, but hostile and unloving women'.[4] While some of these early reports recognised some fathers as highly authoritarian, no connection was made with wider social structures or enabling mechanisms. Further, 'dysfunctional family' models have been offered up as explanations for incest. However, if overcrowding, social isolation, poverty and childhood abuse precipitate incest, why is it predominantly men who are perpetrators? How come large numbers of mothers don't start abusing their sons?

It was only in the 1970s and 1980s that research in the context of second-wave feminism began to challenge assumptions that father-daughter incest was rare, natural or harmless – and to challenge the blaming of victims and mothers.[5] This body of research, drawing on victims' experiences, rejected the dismissals and minimisation as little more than a misogynist attempt to maintain men's power within the family and male sexual entitlement more generally. Incest, therefore, is best understood as an extension of patriarchal relations in the household. It is about men's overwhelming authority in some families to exert control and domination over other family members, including through sexual entitlement.

Examining incest in the context of patriarchy helps us to understand why it is that men perpetrate this abuse more than women.

There are cases of mothers sexually abusing their children, but very few. It helps explain why society listens to men justifying their abuse, denying it or legitimising it. Remember, this is part of a much bigger social structure. It still exerts a powerful influence, but it was of course much stronger in the past, explaining why incest was for so long not properly understood or recognised.

But these emerging explanations were strongly resisted. By the 1990s, feminists raising questions about child sexual abuse were accused of hysteria and the familiar charge of creating a 'moral panic'.[6] But the legitimisation, denials and blaming of mothers and victims had not gone away. A study in 2012 declared that many incest victims were 'not only victims but participants', and that, in some cases, the behaviour of the mother 'could have contributed to the development and duration' of the incest due to 'avoiding sex, emotional unavailability and maternal role abdication'.[7]

What is extraordinary is the effort put in to absolve men of their responsibility for incest. An influential 2017 study is a jaw-dropping example.[8] It talks of 'affection-based incest', and uncritically discusses girls 'voluntarily' engaging in sexual activity with their fathers. Mothers are blamed for withholding affection from their daughters, and it states that the highest predictor for father-daughter incest is 'parental fighting', signalling the 'dysfunction of the parental relationship'. And I am not being overzealous in my reading of this. The research specifically criticises what it calls the 'victim advocacy model', where fathers are held 'responsible' for the incest. The problem is not identified as abuse and coercion by the father, but *parental* fighting. So shifting blame and denial. No analysis of power.

Furthermore, those poor men, in 'problematic marriages to women who are unable or unwilling to provide affection and regular sexual relations', end up turning to pornography and 'risky' sexual behaviours, including extra-marital affairs and prostitution. So now the mother is responsible not only for the sexual abuse of her daughter but also for the husband's affairs and engaging in prostitution. These researchers call their model and approach 'humanistic' and aim to keep the nuclear family intact. They state that 'separation of the father and the daughter is not necessary for treating affection-based incest'.

This is not an isolated example. A 2024 study investigated the causes of incest and said that, when the mother of the victim is 'unable to satisfy the father's desires', fathers 'may seek alternative and tragically more accessible means by placing their desires against their daughters'.[9] A breakdown in relations between mothers and daughters was further said to be causative. How do we avoid this? Girls, it's up to you. The researchers said that it was important for girls to 'maintain a strong bond with their mother' to reduce the 'risk of such issues' arising.[10] These excuses and denials are obscuring the realities of abuse and inhibiting real change.

We know that child sexual abuse is far more prevalent than is routinely acknowledged. It is estimated that at least 500,000 children in England and Wales are sexually abused each year, with at least one in ten children being sexually abused before the age of sixteen.[11] This is predominantly girls – around 15 percent of girls and 5 percent of boys have experienced some form of child sexual abuse – with steep increases reported over recent years.[12] Around one third to one half of these cases are within the family, with fathers and stepfathers the main perpetrators. Of cases reported to the police, approximately two-thirds are perpetrated by a family member or someone close to the child.[13] Though it may be harder to come forward to report a biological father, a Canadian study found that, of the fathers abusing their children, two-thirds were stepfathers who occupied a parental role in the lives of the victims.[14] While some women do commit this abuse, almost all the perpetrators are men.[15] In this context, it's important to note that there is no reported difference in the devastating harms experienced by girls, whether reporting abuse by fathers or stepfathers.[16]

The abuse is carried out in myriad ways. Some involves prolonged grooming, often from an early age, including abuse being justified as 'sex education' and involving pornography to familiarise victims with sexual activity. We can see this replicated in porn videos, where a stepfather is explaining to a young girl the difference between flaccid and erect penises, and she is then seen 'giving' her virginity to him as a 'present'.[17] In addition, it's important to understand that the abuse is across a spectrum and involves rape, as well as actions that wouldn't cross the criminal threshold, such as sexualising the atmosphere with inappropriate comments about bodies or sex lives. These behaviours might also be the precursor to abuse, with girls being encouraged, bribed, tricked, pressured or coerced to take part in activities. These are often situations where control and sexualisation are interlinked. They're often very creepy, uncomfortable, frightening experiences that are difficult to label and understand, especially as a young child.[18]

Finally, while there has long been a reticence to discuss father–daughter incest, there is a deafening silence over sibling sexual abuse. Only recently have we begun to recognise this as one of the more common forms of child sexual abuse.[19] One study revealed that one in ten men reported engaging in sexually coercive behaviour towards a younger sibling during their childhood.[20] In relation to police-reported incidents of intrafamilial sexual assault, one quarter relate to sibling sexual abuse.[21] The most commonly reported pattern of sibling sexual abuse involves an older brother abusing a younger sister.[22]

While these data show staggering levels of abuse, the abhorrent nature of it means that society rarely acknowledges its prevalence; it's more comforting to think of it as something atypical. We don't want to think that all of us will know men who sexually abuse children.[23] However, such myths and assumptions shape the context where professionals are too slow to respond to reports or indications of abuse, often due to high levels of disbelief, where children are not receiving the response needed for their ongoing safety and recovery, where family courts are too slow to intervene, where some judges believe such abuse to be rare and therefore allegations are interpreted as evidence of a mother encouraging children to lie to undermine the other parent.[24]

THE LANDSCAPE OF INCEST PORN

Let's turn then to consider the nature and extent of incest porn. My particular focus is on material portraying sexual activity *between* family members, including stepfamilies.[25] This is where the title of the video, or the story being acted out, involves family members such as 'Slutty stepdaughter secretly wants sex with stepdad'. So the emphasis is not on material where the 'step' label is being used largely as a descriptor for an older man or woman, such as 'aunty grabs the nerdy boy's virginity'.

While the term 'incest' usually refers to biological relationships, I use it more widely to include social families such as stepfathers and stepbrothers, as that is both the reality of families today (and of abuse within families) and reflective of the pornography available. Some object to the term 'incest', largely because it makes us wince. I use it because it conveys the harmful and non-consensual nature of this activity in a way that 'family porn' does not. This is confirmed by the fact that if you search for 'incest' on most porn sites nothing is directly returned, though 'fucked up family' is a searchable category.

In the 1970s, articles in pornographic magazines like *Penthouse* and *Hustler* talked about how the porn industry was running low on taboos being broken, with the time being ripe for a 'new look' at incest.[26] Not content with promoting incest porn though, an article in *Penthouse* argued for a removal of all legal prohibitions on incest, as children were being denied the 'right to sexual satisfaction', with laws criminalising incest 'repressing the sexuality of a lot of children'.[27] These reports tell us first that incest porn was not yet a big thing, but also that the porn industry's drive for something new helps explain the rise of incest porn.

Fast forward to the 1980s and there was still hardly any of this material, only 3 percent of content in one study, where, in fact, there was far more necrophilia.[28] In the first study of internet porn carried out in the mid-1990s, only 1 percent constituted incest.[29] Then, searches for incest porn featuring step-relationships began appearing on Pornhub's list of most popular searches in 2014.[30] The porn industry awards created a new category – 'best taboo relations' – in 2015.[31] By 2016, Pornhub reported that the top three search terms were family-themed.[32] Around this time, many mainstream magazines ran articles about the surge in incest pornography, often discussing incest themes in popular film and TV shows such as *Game of Thrones*.[33] Most trivialised the reality of intrafamilial abuse, preferring a humorous take devoid of any real analysis, though one exception was men's magazine *Esquire*, which rightly stated that it's 'tough to say what the long-term effect of eroticizing incest might have on society'.[34]

To find out more about this kind of content on mainstream porn platforms, my colleagues and I studied the material offered up by the largest three porn sites to a first-time viewer. As discussed before, we found that one in eight titles on the landing pages described sexually violent acts, with the largest category being sexual activity between family members. We only counted titles where there was clearly sexual activity *between* family members, such as 'Brother Fucks Sister In The Ass Outdoors'. This meant we excluded titles that just referred to 'Daddy', 'stepmom' or similar, when they didn't directly connect with other family members. When writing this book, I was really surprised to go back to our study and see that we excluded titles such as 'brother and not sister', which identified the video as a *representation* of family activity, rather than trying to pretend it was a real depition. Therefore, our count is very conservative, excluding much that would now be labelled 'incest' or 'step porn'.

Other studies have found higher levels of incest material. New Zealand research based on the top 200 most viewed Pornhub videos in New Zealand in 2019 reported that nearly half of these featured step or other family sexual activity.[35] They did, though, include all material where the label 'step' was used, which explains their higher findings. They also reported that these videos would often start with the woman actor (as it usually is) initially saying no, but her resistance being overcome by the man's pressure. Any cursory search on the mainstream platforms reveals pages and pages of this material; it's not hidden or niche.[36]

It's important to think not only about the volume of material but also its characteristics: what is it showing? First, there is an overlap between incest and teen porn, in that many of the women actors in incest porn are represented as children through their style of dress and speech patterns, and their appearing in settings associated with children. This is a very deliberate sexualisation of young girls and eroticisation of power imbalances, fostering and emboldening an incestuous gaze. We see this in titles such as 'Real Dad loves his very young daughter', which emphasises the youth, as well as luring in viewers by claiming it's 'real'.

There are many videos that feature actors who genuinely look like they are younger than eighteen. Some of the images continue to haunt me. And even if the actors are over eighteen, the scenes being shown are very clear representations of sexual activity with very young girls, such as a video where the young girl has a dummy in her mouth. Next to it is a video with the word 'pacifier' in the title (the US term for a baby's dummy). That particular actor has her own website showcasing videos of her in a baby's cot. There is no getting away from this as encouraging sexual activity with babies and toddlers.

The images and gifs in incest porn are commonly different from other porn. They are often of just the young girl, her child's clothing, toys and bedroom, and with her vagina on display, emphasising her youth. This is quite a contrast with most other display images, which are anatomical close-ups of penises in the woman's vagina/anus.

Of these scenes involving young/teen girls, there are a few broad themes that play into the denials and minimisation of incest by society and abusers. One is the portrayal of the young girls as seducers and tempters of older men, such as 'I Made Daddy Do

It'.[37] As with mainstream porn in general, the young girls are always available, always keen and therefore always consenting, even if not right at the beginning. Titles suggest that teenage girls want to engage in sexual activity with older father figures. In addition, there's an emphasis on 'first time', 'virginity' and 'deflowering'.

Another theme directly channels more excuses for incest: the mother who is sexually unavailable so the father turns to the daughter, hence 'I am not mom'. We see how the harms are reproduced, with storylines emphasising the sexual activity as a 'little secret' between the father and his daughter. Grooming narratives are common.

There exists aggressive, non-consensual material, with videos including young girls saying 'no'. There are references to 'little' daughters, the fathers 'finally' having sex (the thrill), as well as labels shoring up their power by referring to them 'dominating' their daughters.

Another common scenario is that of the older (step)father/brother surreptitiously entering the young girl's bedroom and initiating sexual activity while she is asleep (aka rape). There is one video that has been viewed 3 million times referring to a father waking up a stepdaughter by initiating sex, as well as similar ones emphasising that the activity is forced, with the young girl struggling and crying.

So take your pick. Your fantasy could be that your step/daughter is to blame for her own violation due to her seductive nature; she's an enthusiastic, complicit participant in the sexual activity. You're helped along in minimising any lurking concern by scenarios sounding playful and fun, such as references to a 'mischievous stepdaughter'. Or you feel the need to justify yourself on the basis of your wife/partner being sexually unavailable. Or she's asleep, and therefore easy to overpower and access, or she's just another body to be forced into sexual activity.

As well as the material between fathers/brothers and daughters/sisters, there is a significant amount of material about stepmoms (and some labelled 'mom'). Gone are the shots of just the young girl's vagina; now there is an older woman seemingly educating the younger man in sexual activity, or initiation into 'true' masculinity, such as 'Stepson becomes man of the house'. This material is generally different from other man/woman porn, as there's less aggression, largely because it's the women who are the initiators. Stepson tends not to spit in stepmom's face, strangle her or call her a bitch. Stepmom is not creeping into family bedrooms forcing sex on very young boys.

It's not only the porn platforms that promote this material; it's easily accessible on X. Together with titles such as 'Daddy's little girl comes home from school; let's now cheer her up', there are user communities of 'incest lovers'. Often, the material is more brazen than on mainstream porn sites, with much being made of the videos being 'real', as well as text describing in detail the videos and their meaning, which is too graphic to repeat here (despite it being on a mainstream social media site).

As ever, Google facilitates all of this, providing an extensive list of websites dedicated to this material following a search for 'incest porn'. Top return is for 'real incest porn videos' with the tagline 'Sex with my real dad'. While you can't search for 'incest' on Pornhub directly, search for it via Google and they return the videos that Pornhub categorises as incest, showing that Pornhub tags it that way to enable swift searches. This commercial drive is evident across social media more generally, with incest being click-bait magic. There are influencers on

TikTok and Instagram amassing thousands of followers after posting about incest, particularly suggesting their relationships are incestuous.[38]

By 2024, therefore, incest porn is being described in the media as 'insanely popular', with one report claiming that, of the most popular 100 videos on Pornhub, 4.1 billion views were for step-incest videos.[39] This includes any reference to step roles, not just those clearly depicting sexual activity between family members, but it still shows the growth in this genre. So, in a relatively short period of time, what was once considered a niche genre with few viewers has now become a dominant fixture of porn.[40] What was once extreme is now mainstream.

As we know from earlier chapters, this doesn't happen by chance. We've seen how the porn industry was searching for new genres, with incest being ripe for marketisation and commercialisation. The companies start making this material, they run adverts for it, people start watching it. It's algorithmically promoted, millions watch it, then millions more want to know why millions watched that video, and so watch it themselves. Before we know it, we're in a vicious cycle leading to more and more extreme incest porn.

This carries on despite the porn platforms declaring their abhorrence of incest porn. XVideos, one of the world's largest porn sites, states in its terms of service that it does not allow material that 'depicts or promotes incest'. Pornhub is the same. What is striking is that these prohibitions supposedly cover the *depiction* of acts, not only real recordings of abuse. Of course, these terms are not enforced, as any glance at their website reveals. They know full well that their terms of service are meaningless, works of fiction, just a public relations exercise. But they continue to claim otherwise, with a Pornhub 'transparency report' claiming that it does not 'allow any content that depicts incest' and that it has removed material violating this policy.[41] This hypocrisy has real effects, with users understandably assuming the material they are viewing is legitimate, acceptable and complying with the terms of service.

We also need to centre an even less palatable explanation for the prevalence of this material: that men are creating and using incest pornography as an outlet for their anger, as compensation for their loss of power and control in their homes and their families, and as a way to push back against progressive societal changes and women's fight for equality. Perhaps this is not necessarily about incest, but about the demise of men's power more generally. This is about how some men may be reacting to the prevailing trends in society, with a sense of sexual power being reclaimed, represented in the ordinary bloke managing to have sex with whoever is close by, including his (step)children and stepsisters.[42] This is exemplified in the comments accompanying some of this material. Next to a video about a father forcing himself on his stepdaughter, one user approvingly commented that 'sometimes you just gotta #MeToo the bitch'.[43]

This is where the overlaps between Big Porn and Big Tech, and the role of male influencers, can be keenly observed. As the explanation for incest itself lies in patriarchy, so too does the rise and popularity of much incest porn. While there is step porn that does not engage with the more abusive incest themes, there is much that does, and more than ever before. It's right in front of us, easily and freely accessible. Incest is about men's power, and incest porn sustains and reproduces that for sexual gratification.

THE HARM BENEATH THE HYPE

Is it a problem that incest porn is so common and popular? Let's start with that argument about direct effects and get it out of the way. When responding to the study highlighting the popularity of 'step fantasy' in pornography, the New Zealand regulator said that this material was 'unlikely to indicate a widely shared desire amongst New Zealanders to engage in sex with family members'.[44] True perhaps, though he did then go on to say that 'it's impossible to know without further research'. So the presumption is that there is no link, though actually we don't know. The suggestion that this presumption should remain until further research is a defence of the status quo, as there will never be research demonstrating clear causal links, as we've learned. Sexual offending is too complex to whittle down to one variable, but fundamentally you will never be able to design and carry out an ethical research study trying to see whether someone viewing incest porn goes on to commit acts of child sexual abuse.

But even if we are saying that there is no evidence of a direct, causal link, this does not mean that there are no implications. First, why are we taking the risk that there is no association? Why are we prioritising the need to view 'daddy fucks daughter' over worries about the prevalence of father–daughter incest and the difficulties of identifying and prosecuting such offending? This returns us to the probability argument raised in an earlier chapter. Does the prevalence of incest porn make it more likely that we continue to have high levels of incest, as well as it being largely ignored across society with victims disbelieved and their harms minimised, than if there was no such thing as incest porn?

The focus must be on understanding how porn influences our sexual scripts and practices. The New Zealand report, having dismissed a direct connection, goes on to identify the incest material as problematic, as it more commonly involves non-consensual behaviour. Furthermore, even when consent is clearly established, the narratives tended to raise 'problematic issues' around power dynamics and 'inappropriate sexual behaviour' within a family context. Somewhat of an understatement.

We see the risks of these sexual scripts in studies of teenage boys that have identified increased problematic pornography use in those engaging in family sexual abuse.[45] We don't know what sort of pornography they are viewing, but seeing as mainstream porn is saturated in this material, it would not be surprising for this to be part of their porn habit. Similarly, the world's largest study of child sexual abuse perpetration found that the use of pornography emerged as a key risk factor.[46]

In addition, the sexual scripts of incest porn are mirroring how this abuse is perpetrated.[47] Survivors have reported on abusers' common tactics, such as capitalising on opportunities when they are alone, raping them in their bedrooms at night, coercing and manipulating them, repeatedly instructing them to be silent and not tell anyone what is happening. These are the exact same sexual scripts replicated in incest porn. Reading survivors' accounts, alongside looking at what is so commonly available on mainstream porn sites, is chilling. As Elaine Craig writes, far from being fantasy, these porn scenarios precisely parallel the factual circumstances of incestuous sexual assault.[48]

Incest porn is particularly insidious in sexualising family interactions. Survivors have struggled sometimes to understand their experiences, as there is often no name for the particular forms of abuse. What do we call it when behaviours have not crossed a threshold of criminality, with no 'obvious' abuse, but a very creepy, sexualised environment? Teenage girls do view porn, often as a form of sex education, to try to understand the sexual world. They're confronted by many things, such as the aggression and violence discussed in other chapters, as well as this family eroticisation. Right there. Normal. Common. Confused, they ask themselves: when this is so normalised, why do I feel so uncomfortable, threatened, disturbed?

It plays out in more ways, influencing men's actions and our subsequent reactions. One of the main ways that men's violence against women and girls is minimised is through strategies of legitimisation, denial and deflecting responsibility.[49] Legitimising is about making it acceptable, understandable, normal. Incest porn, being so widely and freely available on mainstream porn websites and social media platforms, certainly performs this task very well. You can search on Pornhub for your particular fantasy and right next to it is daddy/daughter porn. We become inured to incest, no longer thinking of it as intolerable.

Crucially, as well as the existence of this material on the mainstream porn platforms legitimising it, there's the active and affirming engagement of the users. These are videos viewed millions of times with high approval ratings. Many of these videos are accompanied by users sharing their sexual interest in, and activity with, their daughters and stepdaughters, as well as encouraging and applauding the content in the videos. Some of their statements won't be true; they may not actually be forcing sex on their (step) daughters. Nonetheless, users are gaining a shared sense of this being an acceptable, legitimate sexual interest; they're not actually an outsider, a deviant, a dangerous sexual predator. The participatory nature of mainstream porn today is what is reinforcing and sustaining alarming sexual scripts.

Legitimising is close to denying, as a strategy. Denial involves accepting the existence of the behaviour but giving it a different label. So it's not incest or child sexual abuse, but 'affection-based' incest. Or it's not incest porn reproducing harmful sexual abuse, but fauxcest, fantasy. In truth, even using the label 'incest porn' could be interpreted as a mode of denial. In putting incest alongside porn, seen as consensual, legitimate material, I may be lending legitimacy to incest and casting it in a more consensual light.

Another way to dismiss and minimise abuse is by reattributing responsibility. So if there is any harm in incest, it's not the man's fault. It's the fault of the girls tempting their fathers, of the mothers who are not satisfying their partners' sexual needs. Incest porn is the perpetrator's alibi, helping them deny responsibility and normalise their actions. Even though children cannot legally consent, the prevalence and normalisation of these sexual scripts may subconsciously influence us, the media, regulators, politicians, police, prosecutors, judges, juries.

In these ways, it's not that incest porn directly encourages someone to go out and commit such acts, though it dangerously constructs young family members as legitimate objects of desire. But for those who are disposed towards such activity, incest porn legitimises it and helps them deny their role, transforming intra-familial abuse into a consensual story of sexual attraction rather than sexual violence. Much of it is coercive and exploitative, following grooming scripts where young girls are desensitised to the sexual activity and learn to treat it as normal, though some of it can also be forceful and violent. Studies suggest that the men perpetrating incest are among those sex offenders who most clearly deny or excuse their abuse. Is this because we are providing the environment that makes this easy for them?

WE'RE ALL IN DENIAL

Child sexual abuse in the family environment has thrived in the shadows for far too long. Over decades, this abuse has been excused, casting young girls as temptresses and seducers, with blame placed on mothers said to be neglectful, withholding sex and intimacy. While these ideas originated many decades ago, they continue to resonate. In particular, the very denials and excuses offered by perpetrators are reproduced in patriarchal porn, legitimising them, absolving men of responsibility. This contributes to the enduring tendency to assume incest is rare, to disbelieve reports of child sexual abuse and to minimise the harms experienced. Victims of intrafamilial abuse suffer physical and emotional devastation, and it is troubling, to say the least, that these experiences are eroticised – for profit – by Big Porn and watched by millions.

My concern is about the overall climate that the easy and free accessibility of this material creates and sustains. An individual video is not necessarily harmful (though it might be). But if all we do is focus on each individual post, each individual video as separate, as just about OK, as artistic, as an exercise in the individual right to free expression, we are turning a blind eye to the collective impact. Incest porn normalises incest, distorting viewers' perceptions of family relationships and desensitising us all, with real-life consequences. Incest is not an isolated instance of family breakdown, but is facilitated and legitimised in a wider cultural context where porn in general, and incest porn in particular, plays its part. There is so little attention paid to the connections between incest and incest porn, and when there are public discussions, they are usually of the click-bait variety, musing on the easy availability of this genre of porn, making light of it, as if talking about the latest healthy eating fads.

A significant challenge is that incest is said to be so abhorrent that it's unthinkable, and therefore any representation of it is so fantastical that it's just for entertainment. However, incest porn may be fictional, a depiction, but it is not fantasy. For vast numbers of children, especially young girls, forced sexual activity with their (step)fathers and (step)brothers is very real. It's not rare, it's not unthinkable; in fact, it's common and perpetrated with relative ease. The sexual scripts of incest porn directly reflect the methods of abuse, but not the harms. Far from it. In fact, what we see are depictions of abuse not only being tolerated but celebrated. These are not videos pushing the boundaries of sexual interest; they're not the 'ultimate taboo'. They are banal, commonplace, watched and applauded every day, by ordinary, average men. Part of the porn landscape, incest porn is shaping our porn habits, facilitating and providing legitimacy to rampant levels of intrafamilial sexual abuse and overpowering our social consciences such that we do or care little about it.

8

Without Consent

GIRLS DO PORN. GREAT NAME FOR YOUR PORN PRODUCTION company. Tells it like it is. In reality though, the company should have called itself Girls Get Raped, Filmed and Exposed Online Forever After. True story.

For ten years, until 2019, Girls Do Porn was a small production company in the US that made millions from videos recording the rape, assault and coercion into pornography of hundreds of young women.[1] They deceived the women by advertising for models, only later telling them it would be porn, and then claiming the films would only be distributed to 'private collectors' in Australia. The survivors have told harrowing stories of blackmail, assault, coercion and brutality during lengthy shoots, when many wept, bled, vomited, cried out in pain or begged for the filming to stop.

These videos were never intended to be kept private. On Pornhub, Girls Do Porn were among the most popular videos, clocking up over 672 million views over a period of eight years.[2] This was a popular 'casting couch' genre, with the videos describing how this was the first time these young women were filmed for any adult content: 'This girl was so fucking nervous to do her very first adult video, it took months of convincing to get her to finally agree to do this.' To drive traffic to the videos, the company shared many of the women's full names, contact details and social media profiles online. The subsequent abuse and harassment was off the scale, and continues to this day.

Multiple lawsuits followed. In 2021 Pornhub settled a case in which it was claimed it knowingly profited from Girls Do Porn videos on its platform and failed to stop the videos circulating.[3] Following a federal criminal investigation, Pornhub accepted responsibility for their role in 'hosting videos and accepting payments from criminal actors who coerced young women into engaging in sexual acts on videos that were posted without their consent'.[4] Indeed, despite repeated calls, Pornhub only removed the videos from its site when criminal proceedings were taken against the owners of Girls Do Porn, some of whom have now been imprisoned for trafficking.[5] The videos still circulate, and the abuse continues, aided by cloud services refusing to block this content.[6]

And it's now become even harder to imagine a time when this material will be taken down. It's a new low, wrote journalist Matt Burgess of *Wired*, who has reported many times on the proliferation of non-consensual pornography. In summer 2024, he told me he'd found an account on MrDeepFakes, the largest website dedicated to deepfake sexual abuse, that was using the Girls Do Porn videos as the base material. Deepfakes are where ordinary images are inserted into porn; here the faces of celebrities were being superimposed into Girls Do Porn rape videos. What did I think, he asked? Where to begin. These young women were now experiencing a whole new level of abuse, the video of their rape now being used to abuse other women; their trauma now being repackaged and reshared for a new audience. For the celebrities, not only were their images being used without agreement in porn videos, their images were now being superimposed onto films of rape.

This was no accident. The uploader had a version of Girls Do Porn as his username and included the sex trafficking site in the video titles. As I said in Matt's report, the drive for profit, fuelling the trade in non-consensual porn, appears to know no bounds.[7] It gets even worse. These rape videos are included in some of the bespoke AI databases being used to generate sexually explicit deepfakes, avoiding some of the protections in the general-purpose image generators that any of us might use online.[8] However, even these more legitimate databases may include some of this material, as they've been found to contain child sexual abuse imagery, as well as other forms of non-consensual material.[9]

This is the stark reality. There are hundreds of videos of the rape and abuse of young women that have been viewed and downloaded millions of times. These videos circulate far and wide, being uploaded and shared in dedicated forums across the internet and social media, with communities of users fixated on the videos and the victims, continuing to re-share and re-reveal the victims' personal details. The videos are being used in AI databases to perpetrate yet further abuse. The videos – the abuse – is immortalised online. It's awful to even write this, but these rape videos will never now be out of circulation.

The Girls Do Porn experience tells us much about the industry, the misuse of technology and the seemingly unstoppable desire of so many millions to watch rape pornography. It's nothing new (unfortunately) that men rape women, or that some women help procure the victims (as happened in Girls Do Porn). Not even new that it was filmed for entertainment and profit. What is new is the worldwide reach of Big Porn facilitating the uploading, downloading and constant viewing of this material by millions – and, specifically, an industry prioritising profit over safety, with minimal interest in taking down non-consensual material.

It was not only Pornhub and Big Porn; Big Tech played its role in facilitating this abuse. The payment providers Visa and Mastercard were profiting from these videos being on Pornhub and related websites. Google helped as well, these videos being easily findable via search engines. Multiple forums on social media platforms were distributing links. This is a corporate web and financial ecosystem entrapping these women in a never-ending cycle of abuse.

It further reveals the participatory nature of porn today. Users work hand in glove with Big Porn to ensure the material remains accessible online, to use advancing technology to preserve the videos online forever and to continue modifying them, showcasing rape in new ways for new audiences and keeping the old audience returning again and again. Each step is part of a feedback loop legitimising their actions, making this all seem normal.

I wish I could say that this desire to watch rape videos is unique to this particular case; it's not. I was painfully reminded of this in late 2024, when journalist Adrija Bose approached me about an Indian case where a young woman doctor was brutally raped and murdered when resting in a hospital between shifts. This case was horrific in and of itself, but there was something particular that Adrija wanted to ask me about. In the days following the murder, while there were mass demonstrations and doctors' strikes amid the despair at the epidemic levels of sexual violence, millions of others were turning to Google to search for videos of the rape.[10]

It was not even known if there was such a video (there isn't, as far as we know), but these searchers were hoping to find one. It's so common nowadays to film a rape that there was a high likelihood of there being such a video, or maybe a leaked CCTV recording. They were also searching secure in the knowledge that, if this video did exist, it was likely on a porn site, or Reddit forum, easily accessible. As well as the top Google searches being for the rape video, there were thousands of searches on XVideos with the victim's name.[11]

These are two particularly stark examples of both the demand for rape porn and how it has been allowed to flourish on Big Porn. Unfortunately, these cases are not exceptional. What was once only available on dedicated rape porn websites is now commonplace. And not only in Big Porn, but also on social media such as X.

WHEN RAPE FINALLY BECAME 'EXTREME'

First, let's try to work out how we got here. For nearly twenty years I've been researching rape porn, its prevalence, its harms, what it tells us about society and how it is regulated in law. I've clearly not been very successful in my drive to eradicate it, but that's not for want of trying.

You may remember from the chapter on choking/strangulation that, about twenty years ago, new laws on extreme pornography were introduced. At the time, my colleague Erika Rackley and I pointed out that the definition of 'extreme' did not actually include rape. I went on BBC Radio 4's *Woman's Hour* sharing our concern about the exclusion of websites such as *RapePassion*, which had the strapline 'hardcore pictures and crystal clear videos of young girls brutally violated – 100% forced sex'.

There was a lot of heated public debate about these new measures. Proposing restrictions on access to their porn gets some people seriously riled. One web forum listed Erika and I on their 'Nutter Watch' pages. If 'nutter' was the label applied to those arguing against the eroticisation of rape, then fine, I was happy to be labelled a nutter. That was then; I'm very conscious that the online abuse I would experience today would be far, far worse.

Despite my best efforts, the extreme porn law adopted in 2009 did not include rape porn; it was not deemed sufficiently 'extreme'. However, watching this public debate in England and Wales was Rape Crisis Scotland. They then started a campaign to change Scots law (which is different from the law in England and Wales) to introduce an offence of possessing extreme pornography and, particularly, to ensure it included rape porn. Sandy Brindley of Rape Crisis got me involved, speaking with Scottish government ministers and in the media, making the case for change alongside many others. Unlike in England, the Scottish government was supportive and changed the law in 2010.

England was beginning to look out of step, but change was coming. Fiona Vera-Gray was working in Rape Crisis South London and was hearing from clients about how the rape porn available online was impacting them. She reviewed the most popular rape porn websites easily accessible online and found so much of it being marketed as involving children (e.g. 'schoolgirl rape') and incest, as well as rape involving guns and knives and where women were unconscious or drugged.

Fiona and Rape Crisis did great work getting some internet service providers to block these websites, but they actually wanted to change the law, following Scotland. I worked with them, alongside the End Violence Against Women coalition. Our aim was to raise awareness of the prevalence and harmful impact of this material and, in reforming the criminal law, to make it clear that rape porn should be not viewed as legitimate entertainment.

To support this campaign, Erika and I produced a factsheet on rape porn that we shared with politicians and the public. We described how the websites dedicated to rape porn commonly had banners describing their content and enticing the viewer. One website called *exploited-bitches* had the headline 'nothing is better than seeing these good looking sluts getting raped' followed by telling its viewers that it's 'time to become Tough Guys. Right now.' On the *rape-reality* website the headlines advertised material showing what happens 'when men lose control' and 'enjoy' sex when women are saying no.

Despite this material being easily and freely accessible, we met resistance at first. The government line was that there was no evidence of 'direct' harm, and free speech rights took precedence. We pushed back. I suggested we focus on the fact that bestiality was included in the current law, but not rape. Bingo. This became a front-page headline – that animals were better protected than women.[12] The tide was also turning thanks to the tens of thousands of people who signed an online petition (that was a new thing back then). An extensive coalition of experts and organisations working on violence against women and girls came together and wrote to the Prime Minister calling for change and making clear that 'sexual violence as a form of entertainment causes huge cultural harm'.

So in 2013 Prime Minister David Cameron announced the change in the law, declaring that rape porn was to be banned, as it 'normalises violence against women and girls'. The messaging here was especially important: this was the government accepting our argument that rape porn was legitimising and normalising sexual violence, what Erika and I called the 'cultural harm' of rape porn. We even won support from an influential Parliamentary committee, which endorsed our argument that the new law would enhance human rights, particularly women's human rights, rejecting the 'free speech' defence against regulation. There was kickback. On X I was told to 'slap myself', to stop wasting taxpayers' money and that rape porn would never go away because it is 'good' as 'it teaches discipline'.

This may all sound rather positive (well, aside from the X abuse). Rape porn is recognised for its cultural impacts on society in normalising sexual violence. Human rights arguments are being used to support regulation, and rape porn is finally seen as 'extreme'. A few years after the law was adopted, my colleague Hannah Bows and I sent out Freedom of Information requests to the police to find out how the law was being used.[13] The concerns that the legislation would be used to imprison those practising BDSM were not realised, but we did find that there were hardly any charges for rape pornography. In fact, the vast majority of prosecutions were for bestiality images.

It's not that rape porn is no longer out there. But, whereas ten years ago it seemed somewhat niche and indeed shocking that rape porn websites were easily accessible via Google, it's now mainstreamed in patriarchal porn and on social media like X. What was once extreme is now part of the mainstream. The law may still outlaw rape porn, but its very ubiquity makes the law hard to enforce.

WHAT'S (STILL) OUT THERE?

How do you find rape porn online? A few years ago, you could type 'rape porn' into Google and it would bring up dedicated rape porn websites, as well as links to Big Porn. I pointed this out in Parliament when speaking about the government's proposed Online Safety Bill in 2022. It seems Google did not like these headlines, and shortly afterwards it amended its policy.

I noticed this change when preparing a couple of years later for the workshop with Google executives that I mentioned in the introduction. You'll recall that, on finding rape porn thankfully blocked, I wondered how extensive their new approach was. Not very, it turned out. Yes, they had blocked rape porn and 'forced' porn, but not 'force' porn. I pointed this out to them at the workshop and, not very swiftly but eventually, over a year later, they changed that too.

Maybe this (finally) signals a real change? Maybe now they are more thorough in their approach, committed to actually reducing the ease of access to sexually violent porn? Alas, no. During the writing of this book, I discovered that, while another positive change had been made, 'sleep porn' being down-ranked, they had left untouched similar terms, including 'asleep porn'. Perhaps by the time this book is published, that will have been changed (I recently pointed this out to Google's Head of Human Rights, so fingers crossed).

However, even if that does happen, my concerns about their overall approach remain. It is really unfortunate, but these changes seem performative at best. They are designed to reduce the political heat, rather than make any substantive difference. And even if they were more thorough in the search terms they down-rank, let us not forget that this is just down-ranking. The material is all still there, it just requires some scrolling to reach. Searches for dedicated rape porn websites are still returned, such as *bestrapeporn*, *rapetube* or *rapepornvideos*. I include these website names here so that you can see that they're not difficult to guess, nor would they be difficult to block. One of the websites claims that 'this is just fetish fantasy', and perhaps most of it is acted. Other videos are advertised as 'real rape', though they may be acted and just marketed that way. Whatever the reality, whether acted or coerced, this material is harmful.

These websites host all manner of different rape and force scenarios, such as women being drunk or drugged and then 'forced'. There is a fixation on youth and teens, with one of these websites having a category 'very very young little girl', as well as videos referring to virgins and blood.

These dedicated rape porn websites are deeply disturbing. They are relentless in their glorification and celebration of rape, which is, of course, the point. However, and this is hard to say, while these rape porn websites are indeed truly horrific, their existence is actually less concerning than the material I am about to discuss on Big Porn and across social media. That's because you do have to actively search for the dedicated websites (though it's not *that* difficult, it's not like they're on the dark web). It requires real intent to find these sites; you have to think to yourself, 'I want to see rape porn'. And most of the material is clearly labelled as 'rape' or 'force'. This sexual activity is clearly unwanted, with the women and girls variously in pain, distressed, fearful and/or drugged. The line between consent and non-consent is clear.

What can be worse than that, you might be thinking. The problem with Big Porn and social media sites like X is that the rape porn is even easier to access and thereby legitimised. One recent survey in the US found that as many as 21 percent of men and 11 percent of women reported having seen pornography depicting simulated rape, rising further to 35 percent of men and 22 percent of women when asked about porn where someone pressures another person to do something they did not want to do.[14] Even more concerning is recent research from the English Children's Commissioner, which found that 44 percent of 16–21-year-olds surveyed had seen depictions of rape in porn, specifically when the woman is asleep.[15] This easy availability presents rape porn as normal, acceptable, actually wanted and therefore unproblematic.

We see this most obviously in content where the initial lack of consent is overcome, and the woman or girl then supposedly enjoys it. This not only encourages rape and sexual violence (persevere and it'll be OK), it also makes it more difficult to understand when something is sexual violence or not (it's on X/Pornhub, millions are watching this, it must be normal and OK). This plays out in the lives of real women. Speaking about the prevalence of sexual assault on university campuses, one student recently explained how 'consent is seen as a game and "no" as a tease', and she implicates porn and social media in this lamentable situation.[16]

When we turn to Big Porn, there have been changes for the better, similar to those undertaken by Google, though in a similarly half-hearted manner. Type 'rape' into Pornhub or XVideos and nothing is returned. On Pornhub you get a warning message saying, 'your search could be for illegal or abusive material' and directing you to their 'trust and safety' guidelines.

So rape is not searchable, but 'force' is, which means you get titles such as 'again and again forced'. Pornhub's 'force' category highlights videos that have millions of views, not all with 'force' in the title, but tagged in this way by uploaders and/or algorithms. There are titles about 'crushing' a woman's cervix, breaking her, and anal sex without lubrication being a 'bad idea'. These titles may not technically claim non-consent, but they certainly convey a desire to harm.

XVideos has a category of force that includes one video viewed 25 million times and referring to 'forceful' sex with a neighbour. There's content using terms clearly indicating non-consent, such as getting 'assaulted' when coming home, being 'groped by a stranger', 'molested' by a burglar or held 'captive'. XHamster has a category of 'foced' porn, ready for the moment when 'forced' is blocked but the savvy can still find what they want. If there really was an attempt to reduce the depiction of coercion and non-consent, such content could be easily removed.

There are alternative ways in which non-consent is conveyed and would be (slightly) more difficult to find, such as 'she was already shaking but I wasn't done yet'. But even some of these could be reviewed by searching for 'unwanted' or 'don't', which are common terms, such as 'don't run from me slut'. Another way of saying the same thing: 'a girl who clearly refuses' has four million views on XVideos and is categorised under 'force'. Other videos refer to a 'schoolgirl' being 'ambushed' on a public bus. One video on Pornhub viewed 17 million times refers to a 'struggling slut' fighting off 'rough anal abuse'.

Next, there's content celebrating 'stealthing', where a condom is removed during sex without agreement. This is formally rape, though this is not widely known, perhaps due to its normalisation in media such as porn. There's a film on XVideos, for example, with nearly 4 million views, titled 'Personal trainer took off condom secretly'. Underscoring the inter-relationships between patriarchy and sexual violence, a recent study of stealthing found that men with greater hostility towards women were significantly more likely to engage in non-consensual condom removal.[17]

Other categories of material are similarly non-consensual and depict unlawful activity, but you wouldn't think so from the commonality of them and the almost humorous way they're portrayed. I'm here thinking of the material involving sexual activity with sleeping, drugged or unconscious women, sometimes labelled as 'one-way sex'. Just in case it needs saying, these are deeply harmful forms of sexual violence, with women talking about it inducing hallucinations, flashbacks, extreme hyper-vigilance and real difficulty sleeping, as well as never being able to trust anyone again.[18]

As with the term 'rape', recent (superficial) changes on some of the largest sites make this material initially more difficult to find, but freely available in practice. Type 'sleep' into Pornhub and you get another warning message. This is a recent change, not in place when I spoke with Pornhub trust and safety executives at the end of 2023, when Fiona Vera-Gray and I specifically raised this with them. But by autumn 2024, it was different. This came to light during the French trial of Gisèle Pelicot's husband and fifty other men for her rape while she was drugged. Not only did this case illustrate the extent of drug-facilitated rape, it further raised the role of pornography, as the defendant's internet history included searches for 'asleep porn'.[19] It was claimed that Pornhub had made the change in response to public outrage following the conviction of the men in the Pelicot case.

However, you won't be surprised to know that you can still find all this material. Pornhub still offers up many search options for various forms of sex involving sleep, and you can type 'Pornhub sleep' into Google and it takes you to these sorts of videos. Now it is true that if you removed 'sleep' from all titles, this might eliminate some that are ostensibly consensual, as there are a lot of scenarios involving people having sex while a third person is asleep, such as a partner or parent. But seeing as Pornhub claim that every video is checked before uploading, that would not be difficult. As with Google, is this blocking of just 'sleep' performative, trying to convince us that non-consent and 'trust and safety' is being taken seriously, but without any substantive changes?

Then there's the genre of 'time-stop' porn. This is where the women are frozen in time, as if by magic, so that they are unresponsive and any sexual activity can be performed on them without them knowing or consenting. Hilarious we are supposed to think, just a bit of banter, as clearly there is no spell that can freeze a woman. But there are drugs that have the same effect. Zhenhao Zou plied many women with drugs before raping and filming them when they were unconscious, confirming at his trial that he was an avid consumer of 'time-stop' porn. He said he liked this material as 'the girl appears to be still and quiet'.[20] He shared that he liked 'rape role play' porn. While his conviction was widely reported, there were few mentions of his porn habits and the role that played in encouraging his preferences and behaviours. Nor any discussion of how this type of porn legitimises a sense of entitlement.

This takes me back to the warning page Pornhub returns when blocking searches for rape porn or sleep. Their 'non-consensual content policy' has a specific provision on sleep: 'Where there is a component of sleep in the content, the person must wake up within a reasonable time from the start of any sexual act(s) and consent must be made clear by that person.' I was dumbfounded when I first read this. I couldn't actually believe they'd put this into print. This is a statement permitting rape porn on their website. While rape laws around the world vary, one thing is clear: you cannot consent to sexual activity if you are asleep. No ifs or buts. It's baffling that they have a particular statement on this, suggesting that they know the material is problematic, and so try to justify it. Finally, it's not even the case that all the sleep videos involve the woman waking up after a 'reasonable' time; many involve the woman being asleep the entire time, in others it's a very long ten or more minutes before they 'wake up'.

This matters. While few people read terms of service, perhaps more of them will know that Pornhub has these pop-up warning messages. And the performers and uploaders know that while they are supposed to comply with these terms, they can still upload material in breach. The terms of service give assurance that all the material on the website is consensual and lawful: a veneer of legality. But this is far from the truth and is profoundly damaging in blurring the lines between what is sexual violence and what is not.

RAPE ON X

By now, you know you can find rape porn on X, and there is not even a pretence of content moderation of the word 'rape'. Even though this is a mainstream social media site, the text accompanying these videos is too disturbingly graphic to repeat here. On the most basic of searches, I was presented with an image of a young girl in pyjamas being penetrated from behind with the caption referring to her 'big brother' raping her accompanied by

#rapeme #rapekink as well as various other hashtags referring to incest.

Some users seem worried they'll get blocked, so type r@pe, not realising there is no content control of this material whatsoever. At this stage, it's important to recall our discussion of the business model of Big Porn and Big Tech. Video content, as extreme as possible, keeps users engaged for longer, which means more advertising and more revenue. Pornography on X makes serious profits – that's why it's there, and why there are so few limits.

As with so much mainstream porn, an added concern is the common message that she (always) likes it. Maybe not at first (that's part of the arousal), but persevere and she will. This is a common trope in much aggressive and violent pornography, but on X it's the obvious in-your-face nature of it that is so confronting. This being social media means that the captions and descriptions are lengthier and therefore even more graphic than on porn sites. Coupled with the lack of moderation and therefore blatant racism and misogyny, this means that the nature of the material can feel even more alarming than that found on Big Porn.

The problem is intensified by the rape porn sitting alongside news reports of real rape. You can quite literally scroll through a feed populated by rape porn followed by media reports of rape. Closely intertwined, porn rape and real rape, the same scenarios. Is it any wonder we struggle to identify or take rape seriously when this is the nature of mainstream social media?

Despite widespread concerns about X since its takeover by Elon Musk, it is still one of the largest social media sites in the world, therefore enjoying a veneer of legitimacy, respectability and authority. So the easy availability and brazen nature of this material on such a site lends it similar legitimacy, respectability and authority. It is normalising sexual violence. Yet this is not widely understood.

When I spoke in Parliament about the easy accessibility of violent and misogynistic porn to the group of MPs reviewing the Online Safety Bill, many were shocked when I turned my fire on X. I too had their view of X a few years ago. I knew there was porn on there; I knew that it's one of the first places that young people search for porn. But even I, despite my years of working in this area, thought it was just a bit of soft porn, perhaps directing you elsewhere for the heavy stuff. But, pure and simple, X is a porn site, and one hosting seriously extreme material with inadequate controls.

WHERE NOW?

What I've seen over the years is the mainstreaming of rape porn. While it was deeply concerning all those years ago to have dedicated rape porn websites so easily accessible via Google, that was largely where the material was to be found. It was labelled as rape and clearly unwanted sexual activity, even if it was being created and shared for sexual gratification. But what was once extreme has now morphed into legitimate and normalised sexual activity in mainstream porn. It has the cloak of legality, with the search for rape returning no results, but forced and coerced sexual activity being common and easily available. There's also X hosting content that glorifies rape and rape porn. The reality is that the material and accompanying text that was once the domain of the dedicated rape porn websites is now a staple on X. No labelling, no warning, no need to worry about being seen viewing a website with a title such as *rapedbitch*. Just go on X.

Exposing the reality of X is harder than talking about Big Porn. On one level, few are surprised by what's on the porn sites, even if the extreme nature of it is somewhat of a shock. But when discussing X, I'm often met with a look of disbelief. If the reality does dawn, that look is then replaced by a shoulder shrug: what on earth can anyone do about X? It seems that even regulating Big Porn is easier, and that's true to an extent. Pornhub have at least made some minimal changes.

Yet the stakes could not be higher. Rape porn is playing a key role in making young men think that rejection can and should be overcome, that girls like it even when forced, that coercing someone into sex is normal and acceptable, and that sex with sleeping women is OK.

The rape porn on mainstream porn platforms and across social media actively and consciously confuses our understanding of what is rape and what is consensual, legitimate sexual activity. Consequently, we take rape less seriously. We do not recognise it. We minimise its harms. It creates and sustains the cultural context within which sexual violence thrives, as is so evident in the lives of so many women and young girls.

9

Deepfaked

IN 2017, A MAN ON REDDIT WAS PLAYING AROUND WITH SOME of the latest tech, developing a new algorithm to superimpose someone's face into a video. Everyone had long ago grown used to Photoshopping, but this was new, exciting – potentially a game-changer. This was using the latest AI to make fake, but realistic, videos of someone saying or doing things that they did not say or do. What prompted this desire to develop this new tech? The seemingly unstoppable urge for more porn. This man took images from the web of Scarlett Johansson, Gal Gadot and other celebrities and superimposed them into porn videos. He posted his new creations to his community on Reddit and instantly became a tech legend. In his words, he'd found a 'clever way to do face-swapping'.[1] Very clever, as not only did he give birth to the tech that is now being used worldwide; it's named after him. What was this man's Reddit username? Deepfakes.

Yes, the term 'deepfake', now used to describe all manner of AI-generated videos, in movies and politics, as well as porn, originates from the Reddit forums dedicated to finding new ways to create and share pornography. Not just any porn, *non-consensual* porn. This tech enabled something new, to take a woman's images and insert them into pornography *without their consent*. Deepfakes didn't care. Nor do the millions of men who have since been revelling in this exercise of power over women and girls. If all they wanted to do was see people having sex, they just had to log on; the internet is awash with porn. They didn't need to invent new AI algorithms.

Millions are now visiting websites dedicated to sexually explicit deepfakes and using AI apps to create their own nudes and porn. Many of these sexually explicit deepfakes are of women celebrities. That's where it started, as in the early days you needed a lot of images to develop a realistic-enough video. Scarlett Johannsson was one of the first to be victimised, describing it as 'demeaning', and pointing out that it's ordinary women and girls who will in time be most affected.[2] And that is exactly what has happened, as the tech has become easier and easier to use, with only one photo now needed to produce a non-consensual nude, and with the seemingly insatiable desire to target women and girls continuing unabated.

Miriam Al Adib realised this in 2023, when her teenage daughter told her that the boys in her school had taken one of her photos from social media and made it into a nude.[3] Her daughter was worried, embarrassed, humiliated. But Miriam was having none of it. Her daughter was not the only girl affected in this small Spanish community; the boys were creating nudes of many different girls, some as young as eleven, and sharing them in online groups. They were using 'nudify' apps widely available online and accessed now by millions. So Miriam, a doctor specialising in women's health who has a large Instagram following, spoke out. She refused to let her daughter be shamed and refused to keep quiet. She shared their story, and the world finally began to wake up to the reality of the havoc wreaked by AI-generated 'deepfake porn'. Since then, similar stories of humiliated schoolgirls and enraged parents have been reported around the world, with women teachers similarly being subject to this abuse, fearful for their professional lives.[4]

Sexually explicit deepfakes are being weaponised against women and girls. They are violating, intimidating, threatening, terrifying, demeaning and silencing. The prevalence of sexually explicit deepfakes says to women that their bodies and identities, their sexual privacy and autonomy, are not their own. They are being objectified and sexually harassed on a global scale; they are being silenced and intimidated out of public spaces, with women identifying as LGBTQ+ and Black and minoritised women experiencing higher levels of abuse. To be deepfaked without your consent can be devastating. The humiliation, harassment and abuse are isolating, constant and life-altering. It can be life-threatening, with the weight of shame, abuse and threat feeling unbearable. It can even be life-ending, with reports from Pakistan that a young woman was murdered by her father in a so-called 'honour killing' after a doctored photograph of her with a man went viral.[5] Young women have even taken their own lives following deepfake abuse.[6]

This all started with one man keen to find new ways to make non-consensual porn. It then intensified, as more wanted to join in, with the tech developing incredibly quickly, thanks to the highly motivating urge to create pornography and abuse women. By 2019, a widely reported study found that, of all the deepfakes then available, 96 percent were pornographic and 99 percent of those were of women.[7] Fast forward to today and we are all now part of a society that is generating and sharing millions of non-consensual nudes and pornographic videos.

This has happened with little real concern or challenge. Sure, the mainstream social media companies decry this abuse; and distributing sexually explicit deepfakes was finally made a criminal offence in England and Wales in 2023 and in a few other countries too. But in reality this is now a multi-million-pound business, with millions of users and millions of victims. It is facilitated by the largest social media platforms and payment providers, who advertise apps and websites to produce this material, who enable it to be distributed, who return searches with tutorials on how to make the best videos. Women and girls are bearing the brunt of this new tech, many being victimised as individuals, all now living with the ever-present threat of being deepfaked.

HOW DID WE GET HERE?

It was journalist Samantha Cole who first broke the story of this new tech being created by the Redditor 'Deepfakes'.[8] He was using freely available tech that uses an AI method known as 'deep learning', and what he produced was 'fake' porn: hence his username. While the abusive origins of the term 'deepfake' are sometimes acknowledged, it has mostly been airbrushed out of the tech story, with the term 'deepfakes' becoming commonplace and used to refer to every type of manipulated image or video, not just porn.

Yet these origins are fundamental to understanding, first, why this tech was developed, then why it has advanced so quickly. Porn is one of the main drivers of many technological advances.[9] The rapid development of the original video recorders and DVDs in the 1980s was thanks to porn. Less well known is that a *Playboy* centrefold played a central role in the development of the JPEG file format. For decades, computer scientists blithely used the nude image of Lena Sjööblom as the foundation for their development of image files and processing, caring little about its origins.[10] Twenty years on, some computer science journals no longer allow reproduction of Lena's image. But the reality remains that when the computer scientists were in their lab, working on file formats for images, one of them produced the nude centrefold to use as a test. It just happened to be there, at work, used without challenge and, since then, reproduced thousands of times. All of course without her agreement.

While the first deepfakes were porn videos, this was quickly followed by tech producing non-consensual nudes: what are now called nudify apps, used to undress or 'nudify' clothed images of women and girls. By 2023, these apps were soaring in popularity due to their easy availability in app stores, through being highly ranked by Google, and because they were being advertised across social media sites including TikTok, Instagram and LinkedIn. Some of the statistics are phenomenal. A lawsuit brought in the US against sixteen apps found that, in the first six months of 2024, those apps were visited over 200 million times. We need to be clear: these apps are being used to abuse women and girls. Their software doesn't work on men's bodies, sometimes returning pictures of vulvas, sometimes just blank images. The tech is trained on images of women; it's designed to abuse women.

It is of course possible to nudify an image consensually. But let's face it, that's not what is happening. The millions using these apps are not women and girls uploading their own photos. They know what they look like nude; they have eyes and mirrors. Men and boys are doing this, without women's knowledge or consent.

One of the platforms makes this abundantly clear: 'Imagine wasting time taking her out on dates, when you can just use Undress Ai to get her nudes.'[11] Another emphasises how easy this is: 'see anyone fully naked in seconds'.

Then came generative AI, which produces entirely new images and videos from text prompts, such as a name and sexual activity. This is what happened with Taylor Swift when a group of men on 4chan used Microsoft tech to generate non-consensual sexual images of her that went viral – truly viral, being viewed around 47 million times on X alone. It's important to realise that generative AI produces images using the internet as its source. So it can only generate abusive images, such as those of Taylor Swift, because the internet is saturated with porn. Perhaps even more disturbingly, it can only produce AI child sexual abuse material because there are so many sexual images of children embedded across the internet.

WHAT IS OUT THERE?

The statistics are astonishing, and should stop us all in our tracks. Before it shut itself down (when its owner was about to be publicly named), one of the largest and most notorious sites, MrDeepfakes, averaged around 14 million visits each month. The top forty dedicated deepfake sexual abuse sites had gained 4 billion views by 2023.[12] Similarly, the number of nudifying apps and websites has been spreading like wildfire on social media, with hundreds of millions accessing them. While deepfake abuse began with a focus on celebrities and public figures, men are now targeting the women and girls they know. They are commonly doing this through large communities of online users sharing and trading these images, egging each other on, sharing tips. One investigation of over fifty Telegram groups dedicated to deepfake sexual abuse found at least 3 million users.[13]

No one knows this better than Jodie (not her real name). I first met Jodie in early 2024, during the making of a documentary for BBC Radio 4, when she shared her experience of deepfake sexual abuse perpetrated by a man who, it turned out, was one of her closest friends.[14] He took some of Jodie's ordinary Instagram images and uploaded them to online deepfake abuse forums, asking others to make sexually explicit videos of her. The videos are horrific; one of them is Jodie's image imposed into a video of a young schoolgirl being raped by a teacher. The images were accompanied with messages from the perpetrator saying, 'fake my nasty student … my student makes me so horny' and referring to her as a slut. It wasn't only Jodie. Other friends were being similarly targeted: 'Choose 2 of these sexy sluts I know for a blowjob, and I'll show you more pics of your choice.'

Jodie's experience starkly reveals the reality of this abuse: groups of men online basking in the exploitation of women, bonding together over non-consensual sexually explicit videos, goading each other into producing more and more. And not just any old porn videos, but violent and abusive ones. I'd actually known Jodie for months, working together on campaigns for law reform, before I found out about the exact nature of the deepfake videos. The documentary and media reports didn't talk about images of schoolgirl rape, or anal rape; nor did we. Then she decided to be frank. The government was not prioritising this issue, and Jodie was asked to give evidence in Parliament about her experiences, so she shared the reality of what was in the videos.

Jodie's abuser is not unusual in being part of online communities where men are asking others to make sexual deepfakes for them. Presenter and writer Jess Davies has investigated these groups, revealing just how common they are, with so many men goading each other to make and share sexual deepfakes.[15] The requests are very specific, often deeply misogynistic and often racist in nature (using language that would be condemned if used publicly). Jess provides full details, which include demands for deepfakes of mothers and their daughters, and of men's family members and former teachers – 'would also like the same stuff done to my mum too and would love any edit done to my old school teacher'.

Perhaps it's that the language of nudes, and fake porn, obscures the reality of what these videos are about. Hear the word 'nude' or 'porn' and you don't think of schoolgirl rape, incest or racism. But that's what is being created. Indeed, the first ever deepfake porn video, created by Deepfakes, was an incest stepbrother and sister video. From the very beginning, the nature of the content has been venomous. Search now on these dedicated 'deepfake porn' websites and you can find categories for 'rape', 'rough' and 'incest', just as you can in Big Porn. It's also highly likely that deepfakes targeting Black women will be more aggressive and abusive, as the porn with Black women is of such a nature.[16] In addition, racially minoritised women can be subject to highly politicised and physically threatening deepfakes, such as when actor Mia Khalifa was Photoshopped into an Islamic state execution video following her appearance in a porn scene wearing a hijab.[17]

FAKE IMAGES, REAL HARMS

Helen Mort has written movingly about how, towards the end of 2020, a friend told her he'd found images of her on a porn site: manipulated videos, her face on other bodies, galleries of pictures uploaded by someone who claimed to be her boyfriend.[18] Helen was profoundly disturbed and unsettled. 'I felt violated and ashamed,' she says. 'I was shouting, "why would somebody do that? What have I done to deserve it?"' For a long time, she felt waves of anxiety and fear, and had recurring nightmares of sexual assault by the people in the doctored videos. Helen describes this as a violation of her autonomy, sending a message to women that their bodies and images are not theirs to control, that women can be sexually abused at a whim.

'A picture of an assault'

Helen has described deep psychological harm and trauma. There's the direct impact of the harassment and abuse that often accompanies the distribution of images online. There's the constant vigilance, of wondering who has seen the videos, who is sharing them, where and when are they reappearing. The images included very personal and cherished photographs; one was a graduation photo, of Helen in a favourite dress. That image and memory is now inserted into porn, tainted. If Helen looks at that image now, it 'feels like it's a picture of an assault'.

In one of the deepfake videos, Helen is smiling. It's a holiday photo, now stitched onto the body of a naked woman down on all fours and being strangled by a man. The perpetrator uploaded these holiday photos, pregnancy photos and even pictures of her as a teenager. He encouraged users to edit Helen's face into further violent pornographic photos with the message: 'This is my blonde girlfriend Helen, I want to see her humiliated, broken and abused.' It carried on, 'tell me what you'd do to break my little blonde slut'. Ultimately, Helen says it 'really makes you feel powerless'.

Helen felt haunted; her anxiety increased, picking up her son from nursery became an ordeal as she wondered who had seen the images: she felt on permanent display. Whether you know who did it, or don't, you fear for your physical safety. As with other sexual harassment and assaults, such as being flashed in the street, harm arises through the fear: what might happen next? As Helen says: 'If somebody put all this time into doing that, what else would they do?'

Distrust and dislocation in the world

This all creates a feeling of dislocation in the world. Many women who've had their images taken and shared without their consent describe a deep loss of trust, in friends, family and society generally. Young teenage girls in the US, where boys in their school created and shared AI-generated nudes, speak of their sense of betrayal. They were used to creepy strangers online, but, as one young girl said, 'you'd never think one of your classmates would violate you like this'.

What these girls are experiencing is an awakening to a sense of distrust and despair with those you thought would treat you with respect. It's not only distrust of specific individuals, but a more general sense of distrust of people, of society. It's a sense of unease, of jeopardy. Women's sense of safety in the world has been shattered. Jodie speaks about how the abuse 'undoubtedly altered my view of the world for the worse'. This abuse affects women in different ways, and is especially dangerous for many women in more conservative, sometimes religious, societies and communities. A woman from a South Asian community in the UK has spoken about how 'our lives are already a balancing act of cultural expectations', and that the phenomenon of sexually explicit deepfakes 'just adds another layer, where men will find another way to demonise a woman for something she has no control over'.[19]

Reputational sabotage

We have no control over the sometimes catastrophic impacts on our professional lives, with serious economic consequences. Employers search online when making appointments: who wants to employ the person with a dodgy online reputation, where porn images appear when searching for their name, even if they're fake? US scholar Danielle Keats Citron refers to this as 'reputational sabotage': getting and keeping a job is that much harder when sexually explicit deepfakes of you are all over the internet.[20] Most of us have an online presence of some sort, and for many jobs and professions it's a prerequisite.

Those who make their living online can be particularly affected. Influencer Cally Jane Beech has talked movingly about the devastation of being subject to deepfake sexual abuse and how she lost out financially because of it. People either thought it was actual porn, and so didn't want to associate with her, or they knew it was fake, but still didn't want to work with her as the controversy was not worth it.[21] She is not alone: one investigation found many sexually explicit deepfakes of content creators circulating widely on social media.[22] In the online communities of men trading and sharing this abusive content, there are dedicated categories for YouTubers, influencers and streamers. But it is far wider than employment.

It affects any area of public life, any field of competition – sports, politics, community activities and hobbies – the capacity for reputational, professional and personal damage is immense.

In addition, we must not forget the other women being harmed by the non-consensual creation of sexually explicit deepfakes: the sex workers whose original videos are stolen and used to make this material. These women and men are airbrushed out of the debates, yet it is their bodies that are being shown without their consent, even if the original video was made voluntarily. This is a violation of their autonomy, as well as their professional lives and reputations, a breach of their or the producer's copyright, meaning they lose income. Working in the porn industry is hard enough without also having your rights violated, your work stolen, your role ignored.

Silence: targeting women in public life

This reputational sabotage is particularly intense for women in the public eye. Cara Hunter experienced this punishment for having a voice a few years ago. She was campaigning for re-election to the Northern Irish Assembly. Being a politician is tough in any environment. Being a 25-year-old woman politician in Northern Ireland is even tougher. But it was about to get even worse. Cara describes how May 2022 became the 'most horrific and stressful time of my entire life'.[23] During campaigning, she got a message from a stranger who asked whether it was her in the video. What video, Cara thought. It was a pornographic video falsely claiming to be of her.

She then got messages warning that a video of her had been 'leaked', at which stage she realised people thought it was real, and it had gone viral. She received many really nasty and creepy messages. She was stopped in the street by a man saying to her 'you love it' and asking her to perform a sex act on him. Cara believes this was a direct attempt to intimidate her in the run-up to the election.

Cara was not the first public figure to be directly targeted in this way. In 2018 Rana Ayyub, an investigative journalist reporting on rape, abuse and exposing political corruption in India, experienced a systematic campaign of abuse and harassment that included sexually explicit deepfakes of her being widely circulated.[24] She was in a café with a friend when she was sent a pornographic video with her face morphed onto the body of another woman. She only had to see the first few frames to freeze and throw up. For some, it was obviously a fake. But this did not matter to Rana, nor did it reduce the abuse that followed.

It was terrifying. Her address and contact details were revealed, shared online next to 'I am available'. Her emails and social media were inundated with screenshots of the video, and rape threats were abundant. The effects were physical, her health deteriorated, she could barely eat. Her physical safety was threatened. Her psychological well-being was seriously affected. As Rana says, this was 'slut-shaming and hatred', which felt like being 'punished by a mob for my work as a journalist, an attempt to silence me'. In the end it was no surprise: sex is so often used to shame and demean women, and especially minority women, and especially minority women who dare to challenge powerful men.

This attempt to silence was similarly felt by Kate Isaacs from the survivor and activist organisation #NotYourPorn following a successful campaign to remove non-consensual porn from Pornhub.[25] She became a target on social media, particularly X, by what she describes as a 'small but loud group of men [who] felt they were entitled to non-consensual porn'. They created and shared sexually explicit deepfake videos of her, using footage from a BBC TV interview. They posted her work and home address, commenting that they were going to follow her home, rape her, film it and upload it to Pornhub. Kate says this was 'completely terrifying, I'd never experienced fear like that in my life'.[26] She describes this as an act of sexual violence, profoundly violating, and says that it was clearly meant to silence her.

This is deepfake sexual abuse being used to muzzle and intimidate women in the public eye. It includes sportswomen, having the audacity to excel in sport and therefore deserving to be taken down a bit. It includes women not seeking a public voice but undertaking a public service. A woman doctor giving evidence at a parole board hearing had her testimony turned into sexually explicit deepfakes, which were spread online to diminish her authority and expertise. The message is loud and clear – get out of the public space. Women journalists and politicians already face exceptionally high levels of online abuse and harassment, what the United Nations refers to as 'the chilling': pushing women out of public life and 'chilling' their speech. The effect is particularly marked for Black and racially minoritised women, and women in marginalised and minority groups relating to age and sexual orientation, as well as caste, disability and refugee status. Speaking out about human rights, or women's rights in particular, puts you at an even higher risk of abuse and harassment.

The invisible threat of deepfake abuse
In 2022, Jess Davies made a documentary for the BBC, and its title was striking: *Deepfake Porn: Could You Be Next?*[27] Jess herself has experienced serious online abuse, but she was highlighting that,

not only does deepfake abuse harm the specific women targeted, there is also a collective dimension: it is a threat all women and girls are experiencing. Anyone could be next.

This fear and threat are felt so acutely by younger women. Towards the end of 2023, I was listening to a podcast made by a group of young women students talking about deepfakes and image-based abuse.[28] I was deeply struck by their palpable sense of despair. They talked about how 'all it takes is the unpredictable behaviour' of men to 'knock down absolutely everything we've spent our academic careers working for', and that one 'rash decision by a boy could completely ruin all the progress' that they've made. They spoke about how a woman's reputation is 'so fragile', even though they know that's not how it should be. They despaired at how this 'amazing tech' is being used in this way. It's a 'really scary' threat at the beginning of their professional lives.

I felt this too in my classroom, exploring with students how the law is failing to protect women and girls from deepfake sexual abuse. We talked about how they could be in the lecture theatre, when someone just sitting alongside could instantly make a deepfake of them, tell them they've done so, that they will use that video later, and yet there is very little the women can do. In seminar after seminar, women expressed their outrage and despair. I'll never forget the undercurrent of rage of one young woman, who sat back, folded her arms and said: 'I am so not happy with this.' Total understatement. But what else could she say? Few seem to care.

Ever since, I've tried to raise this issue of what I've called the 'invisible threat'.[29] The prevalence of deepfake tech and sexually explicit deepfakes have created an embodied sense of unease in young women and girls, on top of the ever-present threats of sexual violence and of street harassment. We might think this is not the worst of the harms in the world. But we must not ignore what women and girls are internalising.

We are used to negotiating and managing, every day, the risks and threats of men's violence. We make active, and often unconscious, decisions about where to walk, where to sit on public transport; we humour the taxi driver who's being a creep because we just need to get home safely; we ignore the shouts of 'cheer up' or 'smile'; we remember to cover our drinks when out (or throw them away and have to buy another if we forget). The list goes on. Fiona Vera-Gray has talked about how women have to hone and develop just the 'right amount of panic' to navigate and manage our daily lives.[30] In the context of street harassment, Fiona writes about how women trade freedom for safety. What we are now seeing is this burden being felt in additional new ways. We are trading freedom online for safety and protection from harassment and abuse.

So many women have talked about how their experience of online abuse has affected their online lives. Women have told me that returning to social media after this sort of abuse is an entirely different experience. They come off certain social media sites, perhaps the ones where the abuse started. They share less, they use social media less.

The difference is that, for people who've not experienced this abuse, the phone in our hands represents a pleasurable activity; it can be a break from work, from the world, to scroll through a few funny videos, recipes or family updates. But for those who've experienced abuse, the phone becomes a site of trauma. Every time they pick up their phone, they're worried there will be another abusive comment, another message saying their image has been shared, another reminder of what is out there. Tech is no longer empowering or an enjoyable social activity; it's a necessary evil.

WHEN THE FAKE BECOMES REAL

I've tried to explain the devastating impact of deepfake sexual abuse because it's still not fully recognised, often due to an assumption that, as it's 'fake', there's no real harm. The creator of the website MrDeepfakes told Jess Davies in her documentary: 'I think that as long as you're not trying to pass it off as a real thing, that shouldn't really matter because it's basically fake … it's a fantasy, it's not real.' Unfortunately, his view is shared by many.

However, for survivors like Helen and Rana, whether the image is seen as 'fake' or real doesn't make a difference to the harm suffered. We know fake news travels faster than real news. It's more thrilling, lurid or divisive. Study after study shows that we are useless at identifying deepfakes; we think we can do it, but we really can't. Then the algorithmic preferences of social media highlight the extreme (more likely false), and our cognitive biases mean we have an understandable predisposition towards certain stimuli, like sex, gossip and violence. This is a breeding ground for the viral distribution of sexually explicit deepfakes, even if someone, somewhere is trying to shout above the noise that it's digitally altered. Any debunking of the fake will come too late and, in any event, it won't alter how women feel about the videos made of them without their consent or the impact it has on their lives. For victims, the images 'feel real'; they are actual images on people's phones, on the internet, except they are altered images.

This is why I think we need to change our terminology and call this material 'sexual digital forgeries'.[31] This emphasises the false nature of the images: it's stealing someone's likeness and sexual identity, creating a false representation. The term 'forgery' clearly labels this as fraudulent and unlawful behaviour. This term was first developed by Mary Ann Franks and Danielle Keats Citron and is used in US legislation on deepfakes, in Council of Europe guidelines, as well as being increasingly adopted by campaign groups.

This is a more adaptable term, to be applied to all manner of abusive content that is being developed, beyond deepfakes, such as the sexual use of avatars of easily identifiable real people. We will soon be seeing this in augmented reality tech incorporated into our everyday lives. This is where 3D experiences are integrated into existing 2D tech, such as augmented-reality glasses that display satnav directions, allowing you to walk down the street with the navigational directions superimposed onto your surroundings in front of you. Translate that into porn, and you might be having sex with someone, but augmented reality tech overlays an image of someone else over your partner's face or body. So rather than you just dreaming of having sex with someone else, you can see them superimposed on top of your partner.

Not surprisingly, augmented reality has much darker applications. At the end of 2024, a group of male Harvard students adapted Meta's 'smart' glasses to enable them to reveal the personal information of people nearby in real time. Known as 'doxing', sharing such private and personal information poses significant dangers, including facilitating stalking. While the creators defended it as a straightforward combination of existing technologies, their lack of acknowledgment of its harmful implications was alarming.[32]

My immediate thought was that next they'll integrate nudifying tech into the glasses so that you can walk down the street, or sit on the bus, wearing smart glasses that nudify the women and girls in front of you. It's almost certainly being developed at the moment.

WHAT'S THE FUTURE?

The underlying problem is that women's sexuality is policed in a way that is simply not the case for most men. There is a gendered stigma around nude and sexual images, meaning that if they are created and shared, the adverse impacts on most women are far greater than if images of men are shared, though young teenage boys are particularly targeted in sexual extortion scams, with often devastating results. It's further reliant on a disregard for sexual consent. Ultimately, to make a difference, we need to live in a society where men do not want to create and share non-consensual porn; where young boys know, just know, that you don't create and share sexual images without consent, in the same way that they don't walk out of a sweet shop without paying for the sweets. This, then, is about more than just regulating pornography and online abuse. It's about nothing less than ending patriarchy.

When Samantha Cole first wrote about deepfakes in 2017, her article was headlined 'AI assisted porn is here and we are all f*cked'.[33] She was so right, yet few of us listened, and even fewer acted. There is now an epidemic of deepfake sexual abuse. Small steps are being taken to bring about change. Some countries are introducing criminal laws. Some platforms are removing access to some search terms and removing some apps. Some countries are introducing some attempt to regulate internet platforms. But there is, in all reality, no real urgency, no real understanding of how this impacts women and girls.

What started in 2017 as individual computer (and porn) enthusiasts developing tech has become a fully fledged, multi-million-pound online industry, with advertising on mainstream social media such as Instagram, X and LinkedIn, propped up by the payment providers. To be clear: this is not all on the dark web. It's easily accessible and right in front of us, just one click away via Google and other search engines. Deepfake sexual abuse is making significant sums of money for many people, including the largest social media and search platforms, and there seems little likelihood of real change.

10

Virtual Realities

PORNHUB MAKES A LOT OF MONEY FROM ADVERTISING, AND IT seems there are few limits on what it will promote. Consider this advert for the 'newest sex simulator game', where you can 'fuck your stepfamily members'. You get to 'control the actions, scenes, positions', with the invitation to 'immerse yourself and feel the real sex experience rather than just watching normal porn'.[1] This is virtual reality, but what is being sold is 'real' sex. This is not just watching porn; you are in it. And it's the next big thing.

Virtual-reality porn is touted as more arousing, more intense. It's even supposed to make us more empathetic. No wonder the porn industry is investing millions. It's the fastest-growing porn sector, and while it comprises less than 5 percent of the adult industry at the moment, this is set to rise to 50 percent by 2030.[2] Big Tech is investing billions in what it calls the metaverse. This is the next iteration of the internet – a virtual world where we will all be living our social, educational and professional lives, maybe conducting business, managing our finances. We won't be having Zoom meetings in 2D, we'll be in virtual environments, experienced through our avatar – our digital twin. This is the 3D 'embodied internet', where you are 'not just viewing, but doing'.[3] You might have first heard of the metaverse when Facebook rebranded itself Meta in 2021, signalling where it sees the future.

Like most tech, the rapid development of the metaverse and virtual reality is being driven by porn. A classic example is Meta's introduction of a 'lying down mode' for its virtual-reality headset. It says this is for comfort and mobility. Sure. It's known online as 'masturbation mode'.[4] And while Apple first tried to prevent porn being used on its virtual-reality headset, it didn't take long for workarounds to be found and shared online.[5]

Now if all this sounds niche, not something to worry about, think again. While virtual reality has long been associated with gaming, it extends far beyond this, permeating many aspects of our lives, not least the development of the metaverse: though I would note that gaming platforms like Roblox boast over 88 million daily users.[6] A recent study from the US found that one third of teenagers have virtual-reality headsets.[7] In the UK, stats from 2022 show that one in fourteen young people were using virtual reality each week, a figure that is only going to have increased since then.[8] In relation to porn, 15 percent of men have watched virtual-reality porn, increasing to one in three men who own virtual-reality headsets. Not surprisingly, most virtual-reality porn users are men, and most are under thirty-five years old.[9]

I want to introduce you to the world of virtual-reality porn, looking into how some of this technology is currently being used, and what this might mean for the future. I want to puncture the idealism around this tech, challenging the PR that this will be more empowering, more arousing, making us more empathetic, despite everything we know about the porn industry. Mostly, I want to examine this growing field from the perspective of those who are most likely to be on the receiving end of the adverse uses of this technology: women and girls.

WHAT IS VIRTUAL REALITY, AND WHO IS USING IT?

There are different ways to engage with virtual reality. We can still look at 3D images on a flat screen, such as our computer, TV or phone. This is how most of us will first encounter virtual reality, how many enjoy gaming, and how you use virtual-reality porn on the major porn platforms. But the real deal is when you put on a virtual-reality headset and become immersed in another world. This can be part of a standalone game (and that includes porn games – yes, they are a thing), or you can enter virtual-reality worlds such as the metaverse.

The first key point to understand about being in virtual reality is that it feels real. This is the masterstroke of this technology. It doesn't matter that we know we're wearing a headset, perhaps standing in our living room. It feels as if we're really in the virtual-reality world, at a rock concert, in a supermarket, in a meeting or in a bedroom with a porn actor. The brain is tricked into this in very clever ways that are difficult to understand until you're in it. This is, of course, the whole point of the tech. The full-sensory, physical nature of virtual reality and the metaverse means that it is experienced as intense, as visceral, as hyper-realistic.

When wearing the headset, you feel like you are 'inside' the scene rather than just watching it on a screen. The virtual-reality environment responds to your movements, tracking your head as you look around the scene in any direction. You physically move when someone comes close to you, as it feels as if they are about to touch you; you might stand on a cliff edge so you don't step off, as it feels dangerous. It feels like the porn actor is walking towards you, whispering in your ear, looking into your eyes, sitting on your lap and touching your body. It's a physiological, embodied experience. This is why some people suffer motion sickness when in virtual worlds, as their bodies struggle to process what's happening (with women being worse affected, as the headsets are not designed with women in mind).[10] So when people say virtual reality is not 'real life', this misunderstands the nature of the experience. It is real, you are in it and doing it. Virtual reality is genuine reality, it's just a different reality.[11]

There is more. What makes this tech transformative is that it also involves touch. You are not separate from this virtual world, but physically engaged in it. As well as the headset, there are devices including gloves, vests and even full-body suits that vibrate or apply pressure in response to the action in the virtual world. These haptic technologies, as they're called, do have amazing potential, such as in medical contexts, where it's used for virtual breast examinations to detect cancer.[12]

However, this is porn we're talking about, and there's a burgeoning sex-tech market selling you wearable kit. These are smart sex toys, called teledildonics, that can be synchronised with virtual-reality experiences, in real time. Let's be blunt: this means devices attached to the genitals so that your virtual-reality partner, an avatar in a scene or another person operating their avatar, can pleasure you. A man may wear what's called a 'fleshlight' (which automatically strokes the penis in sync with action on screen), as well as there being dildos, butt plugs and all manner of other devices.

With haptics and sex tech, you are truly part of the scene. Conventional porn is passive, you are watching it; but with virtual reality, you actively participate, giving a sense of agency. You can 'reach out' to touch or interact with virtual characters and be touched back, making the experience personal and unique. A further aspect to understand is that, in virtual-reality worlds, you very quickly start to identify with your avatar – your virtual twin. While the options are almost infinite, we tend to create avatars very much like us: same gender, ethnicity, hair colour, style. Our avatar doesn't represent us, it becomes an extension of us; it is us. It's this immersion, intensity and embodiment that amplifies the emotional and psychological effects of virtual-reality pornography.

There's also the disturbing world of cyber-brothels, where AI, virtual-reality porn and sex robots combine to provide a whole new way of experiencing porn and virtual/robot sex. Writer Laura Bates describes in horrifying detail how this tech enables users to participate in virtual-reality porn at the same time as physically interacting with a sex doll. The characters offered up for this experience include 'stepmother', 'submissive Yuki', 'Asian Lili' and 'schoolgirl'. As Laura asks, are alarm bells ringing yet?[13]

IS VIRTUAL-REALITY PORN MORE AROUSING?

If it's so immersive and intense, is it more arousing? According to Pornhub, viewers of their virtual-reality porn spend two minutes less time on their site, and they imply that this is because they orgasm more quickly.[14] But the real pull, where the market and technology is developing fastest, are the possibilities of customising virtual-reality porn to your own preferences and tendencies:

no blocked search terms like rape and incest in this virtual world. You choose the setting, the sexual activity, your partner. You can have virtual sex with a celebrity, your favourite porn star, maybe you generate a realistic representation of your ex-partner, colleague, neighbour, stepdaughter. And this is what makes it such a tantalising prospect.

The industry hype is buoyed up by several studies suggesting virtual-reality porn increases sexual arousal. One study compared men and women's reactions, discovering that men found virtual-reality porn more arousing.[15] However, the women did not, with reasons not hard to find. The porn came from Pornhub, which very kindly provided its premium content for free to the researchers. No surprise, therefore, that women did not find the patriarchal porn from Pornhub more arousing. While the authors state that Pornhub was not involved in the research analysis, it's evident that the platform anticipated a commercial advantage in supporting the project; why else would it hand over its material for free? As ever, Pornhub's PR instinct was right, and positive news stories have flowed about virtual-reality porn being more arousing. But note, there were no headlines saying the women were unimpressed.

Another large virtual-reality porn platform, VirtualRealPorn.com, will have been similarly pleased by the results from a study they supported by supplying their premium products for free (and their website is helpfully hyperlinked in the article).[16] The researchers found that, compared to traditional porn, men watching virtual-reality porn reported feeling more aroused and desired, as well as more 'flirted with' and connected to the actors. The researchers declared virtual-reality porn to be an 'empathy machine'. Sounds great. But what was absent from this study?

Women. They're not the only ones who forgot about us. Yet another study sourced its materials from a large, mainstream provider, this time DaboinkVR, and they only studied men. Surprise, surprise, they found the men liked the virtual-reality porn.[17]

So far, we know that men like porn and that they really like virtual-reality porn. But that's not all we found out from these studies. Thankfully, we got an answer to the burning question of whether fifty 'healthy' men thought women actors in virtual-reality porn were more intelligent than those in conventional porn.[18] Turns out they think women actors in virtual reality had higher IQs. I think we learn more here about the men's IQs.

These researchers, and the porn platforms, have a lot to learn from a different study. This one didn't take free material from the largest porn companies but sourced their own virtual-reality content, avoiding depictions of degradation and violence, and from production companies focused on women's pleasure and ethical practices. What a difference. Women did find this content more arousing than conventional porn.[19] However, the researchers speculated that this might simply be due to the rarity of women's perspectives in mainstream porn, making this a novel experience. So change the porn, and you might just change women's reactions.

IS VIRTUAL-REALITY PORN REALLY AN 'EMPATHY MACHINE'?

As well as being more arousing, we are supposed to believe that virtual-reality porn is an 'empathy machine'. This debate all began about ten years ago, when a virtual-reality filmmaker talked about virtual reality as the 'ultimate empathy machine' in a popular TED Talk.[20] He suggested that, through virtual reality, 'we become more compassionate, we become more empathetic, and we become more connected. And ultimately, we become more human.' The technology itself, he declared, regardless of content, possesses an unparalleled capacity to create an empathetic connection, offering a more direct way to enter another person's lived experience, bringing us closer to what cinema, theatre, literature and other artistic media have attempted in the past.[21] This is similar to the findings of journalist and documentary-maker Nonny de la Peña, sometimes referred to as the godmother of virtual reality, who uses virtual reality to create stories, which, she says, 'you remember with your entire body and not just your mind'.[22]

There is some truth in all of this. Positive impacts can be seen in some 'immersive journalism' that brings to life the reality of being a refugee, a person with disabilities or an individual experiencing racial discrimination.[23] We can also see virtual reality being deployed with varying degrees of success in domestic abuse perpetrator programmes, in awareness-raising campaigns about street harassment, and as a tool for caregivers to better understand the experiences of their elderly clients.[24] It is not always going to produce positive outcomes though, with some research suggesting that, rather than building empathy, it can actually have the opposite effect.[25]

Translated into porn, the idea is that virtual reality encourages greater connection with porn actors.[26] It's similarly said that this kind of immersion could demystify sex work, humanise performers, challenge stereotypes, reduce stigma around non-traditional relationships and help users understand sexual preferences or experiences different from their own.

However, the idea that virtual-reality pornography functions as an empathy machine is deeply flawed. First and foremost, the primary purpose of virtual-reality porn is not education or emotional connection – it's arousal. Pornography, by its nature, prioritises fantasy and performance over authentic representation. This creates a fundamental tension: empathy requires authenticity and emotional engagement, but virtual-reality porn is designed to cater to the user's particular desires, often at the expense of realistic portrayals.

Moreover, such porn risks reinforcing, rather than dismantling, harmful stereotypes. Instead of humanising performers or promoting understanding, it is far more likely to amplify existing power dynamics or objectify individuals by reducing them to customisable digital experiences. This comes from the very detailed specification of virtual reality where users may feel a heightened sense of control over performers or scenarios, likely entrenching entitlement rather than fostering empathy. Indeed, one virtual-reality porn site claims that its games 'can make you feel empowered' (though perhaps 'entitled' is a better description).[27]

At root, empathy requires context, reflection and dialogue. While someone might briefly experience a different perspective, they do so within an idealised, hyper-sexualised environment that does not mirror the complexities of real life. Research also consistently shows that we tend to empathise more with those who are like us.[28] It seems unlikely, therefore, that the standard user of virtual-reality pornography – young, high-income men – are likely to become more empathetic towards women sex workers, or the rest of us, by virtue of a more realistic experience of their sexual fantasies that tend to subjugate us.[29]

The promise of virtual reality to democratise empathy across diverse social lives is at odds with how we typically behave.[30] It seems unrealistic to imagine that virtual-reality pornography would generate empathy for others when it is so quintessentially about the users' own needs and ends. Moreover, it reveals something deeply troubling about our society that we are hoping that fancier technology is going to improve our human connections.[31] Indeed, the evangelists of virtual porn seem to ignore the studies on empathy which acknowledge the power of non-technological activities, such as reading about others, to increase empathy, and find that virtual reality is not more effective at doing so.[32] Some suggest that, in actual fact, instead of generating empathy, virtual reality and AI may impair our capacity for empathy, as we are so engaged in the tech rather than with individuals.[33]

VIRTUAL EXPERIENCE, REAL CONSEQUENCES

While I don't doubt the capacity for virtual reality to sometimes foster greater understanding of other people's lives, or indeed that it might be more sexually arousing for some, it's the lack of attention to the likely misuses of the technology that is (as ever) so concerning.

We seem to have learnt nothing from the early incarnations of virtual reality, such as Second Life, where the free-for-all ethos empowered users to adopt child-like avatars, with as many as one in five engaging in what some call 'age play', but which should be called out as simulated child sexual abuse.[34] No surprise, therefore, that one easily accessible virtual-reality app includes the 'game' called 'Let's Play with Nanai', a character described as an adult, but the inclusion of school uniforms and classroom settings suggests otherwise.[35]

In virtual worlds, simulated sex with child-like avatars may involve real children, as there are few controls limiting access to the metaverse and other virtual worlds. Reports are increasing of immersive online environments like the metaverse facilitating and encouraging child sexual abuse both through grooming and interaction with real children, as well as simulating sexual activity with child-like avatars.[36] Even if this involves adults role-playing, it has serious implications for real children by reinforcing and legitimising men's sexual interest in children. Research with contact and non-contact child sexual offenders increasingly finds what is called 'cognitive distortion', where offenders believe that the virtual space is not 'real', allowing some perpetrators to justify child sexual exploitation because their actions are not physically harming actual children.[37]

As well as customisation involving children, the ability to tailor virtual-reality porn creates opportunities to produce sexual scenes involving known individuals, perhaps a user's ex-partner, neighbour, colleague or stepdaughter. While these are different from the deepfakes I talked about in the previous chapter, which are realistic –it really does look like an authentic video or image of that person – the avatars and other creations of virtual reality, while not realistic, can still very clearly resemble a known individual.

On forums such as Reddit, marketplaces such as Patreon and on standalone websites, communities of anonymous users are making, selling and masturbating to computer-generated likenesses of celebrities and other real people. The 3D models that emerge from these communities can be manipulated in ways that defy the constraints of physical reality and interacted with in real time. This means an avatar of some shape or form that looks clearly like an identifiable individual, and you can make them perform your chosen sexual acts. The user is engaging in sexual activity with a very obvious representation of a particular person.

One man reported doing this to 'fulfil my sexual fantasies or replicate sexual encounters with my ex-girlfriends'.[38] The user was specifically talking about a programme that uses a photograph of a real person's face to automatically generate a 3D model with the same face, which can then be used in virtual reality. Another said that this tech enabled him to 'feel like I'm there again, getting a handjob/footjob from my ex looking at me with a smile, or having another ex ride me on the floor in reverse cowgirl in front of a mirror ... the possibilities are endless.'[39]

This is one step beyond creating a deepfake video of someone and watching it for sexual arousal; this is creating a virtual person that closely resembles a specific individual and having sex with them. It is active sexual engagement, using sex tech that provides physical sensations, without that person's consent. These creations and interactions can also be recorded, then shared online, so more people can either view the video or use that virtual reality avatar and interact with them sexually. Just to be clear, this means that someone might create a realistic avatar of you in virtual reality and then share that online for an infinite number of others to comment on and use for their own sexual activity. This is non-consensual sexual activity on a whole new level. I am already getting reports from women that this is happening to them, with one woman sharing that an acquaintance had created an avatar of her engaging in sexual activity and shared this online. She reported it to the police, who said there was nothing they could do about it. (It's true, there is no criminal offence specifically covering this conduct, but it could amount to harassment or a communications offence.)

This is happening and spreading due to the participatory nature of today's porn world. Just as the first deepfakes came out of online communities where men were competing with each other to produce and share the latest non-consensual porn, so these AI and virtual-reality developments are spawned from online communities on platforms like Discord and Reddit, where communities exchange ideas, technologies and custom-made characters. Big Tech and Big Porn are investing billions, but they do so knowing there are vast communities desperate for their products, as well as effectively co-producing the tech advances. Virt-a-Mate, for example, was developed through crowd funding, first launching in 2017 and still going, allowing users to create realistic, interactive avatars.[40] These peer-support networks lower any inhibitions or concerns about the ethical implications of what they're doing.

While some claim virtual-reality porn will be a more humanising and less objectifying form of pornography, there's little to suggest that it will be any different from conventional porn. The experience to-date of the virtual worlds being created and the AI products we are all increasingly using, is that, when existing inequalities are not acknowledged or addressed, they tend to be replicated and augmented in virtual realities.[41] We tend to make new worlds based on who we are and what we do in old worlds, meaning our design choices tend to replicate what we know. This is particularly so when being done at speed and in a high-pressure commercial environment. The adverts on Pornhub for customisable stepfamily virtual-reality porn is an obvious example.

The individually curated material is also likely to reflect current forms of pornography, with the risk that, without the current (minimal) controls on conventional porn, more abusive or violent material is produced.[42] The market for sex robots, for example, does not augur well, where dolls with personalities such as Frigid Farah are designed to reject sexual advances, encouraging the user to rape her.[43] Further, the site Sex Emulator tempts users by encouraging you to 'build your own perfect girl in porn games and fuck it'. 'It' – not a typo – is how they refer to the customised avatar. True, it is a thing, an avatar, but this phraseology feels as if it conveys a lot more. The site continues, stating that it 'lets you train your wonderful woman in all kinds of nasty but useful sexual skills', and 'where everything is customizable and the only limit is your own imagination'. What would you want your 'dream girl' to do? The site suggests activities such as 'ruthless gangbangs, getting fucked by a dozen black guys at the same time'. This doesn't sound like virtual-reality porn as an empathy machine. Nor is it 'setting the sexual imagination free', as some have hoped.[44] It is amplifying everything harmful about mainstream porn.

THE FALSE PROMISE OF VIRTUAL REALITY

The real risk with virtual-reality porn is that any extreme, degrading or abusive scenarios become all the more intense, real and arousing. The boundary between what is authentic and what is on a screen is reduced, and the feeling of actually doing it, being there, is much stronger and more intense. More than ever before, it really does feel like you are forcing a woman or a very young-looking girl to have sex with you. I'm concerned this will strengthen the sexual scripts being played out; they will become more embedded in our thinking and behaviours due to the immersive, intensive nature of the experiences. If this were lovely, empathetic porn where we understood each other more, connected with each more on a human level, it might be good. But that is currently niche and likely to remain ever so. This is the same old porn in a new guise. It will not only intensify arousal, but also likely intensify the reproduction of harmful sexual scripts, entrenching patriarchal entitlement and values.

The hype and idealism around virtual reality generally, and virtual-reality porn in particular, is a dangerous comfort blanket for the industry and everyone participating in it. As ever, we seem to have learned nothing from our earlier experiences of technology. Despite growing awareness that social media actually leads to human *disconnection*, we seem to think that this tech will make a difference. Or, rather, Big Tech and Big Porn are managing to convince us – yet again – that their products will positively transform our lives. Transform, yes, but not necessarily for the better, and certainly not for women and girls. Just as social media has made many of us more isolated, in all likelihood, the supposed empathy and connection felt in virtual worlds will be fleeting. When the headset comes of, the offline world becomes ever greyer, leading to greater disconnection, disempowerment and disengagement from the world. It will be loneliness, sadness and abuse that becomes more intense and more common.

11

How We Fight Back

In 2018, actor and musician Chrissy Chambers achieved a landmark victory in the fight against non-consensual pornography. Years earlier, her then boyfriend had secretly recorded them having sex and uploaded the videos to multiple websites without her knowledge. There wasn't a specific law covering what we now know as image-based sexual abuse, then called 'revenge porn', and the police showed little interest in pursuing any other charges.

With the criminal justice system failing her, Chrissy and her legal team turned to an innovative strategy: leveraging the civil law. It took a few years of legal battles and negotiations, but a settlement was agreed, with some significant wins.[1] Chrissy's ex-boyfriend was ordered to pay her damages, and, crucially, the copyright in the videos was transferred to her. She was able to take back control of her image and identity, using copyright law to insist the videos be removed from social media and porn sites.

Like so many victims of sexual violence, Chrissy wanted to use her experience to help reduce other women's suffering. We spoke together at an event in 2015, when she was one of the first to openly share the devastating nature of this newly emerging form of abuse, and I called for law reform to recognise women's experiences.[2] While Chrissy's case was a breakthrough, the outcomes she secured are unfortunately still rare. It's little known that you can use the civil law against perpetrators, largely because you need specialist lawyers, and that's expensive. But it's an avenue that should be opened up for everyone. I set out in this chapter how we can make that ambition real, as well as sharing suggestions for strengthening the criminal law, and better holding Big Porn and Big Tech to account. The porn industry itself is also a focus, particularly how we might improve support for those working in the business, as well as enabling the production of more ethical, indie porn.

TAKING BACK CONTROL

Usually, the first thing that someone wants to do when they find out their intimate images have been shared online is to get them taken down immediately. The criminal law doesn't help here, however, as it's designed to hold offenders to account for what they've done, often years later, rather than to provide an instant remedy. While there are support organisations such as the UK's Revenge Porn Helpline doing phenomenal work on a tiny budget to get content removed from the internet, we need legal avenues available to all victims *as of right*.

This is where civil law reform comes in, and it's about victims reclaiming control of their lives and images. As we saw in Chrissy's case, it is possible to go to court to get damages against someone who has harmed you, as well as orders to stop the spread of non-consensual imagery. You can even get an order preventing someone from distributing material if they're threatening you. Chrissy also got copyright transferred to her, as did victims of the Girls Do Porn trafficking ring discussed in an earlier chapter.

So the current law can work for some people. A more recent example is a woman who sued her ex-partner for filming her without her consent while she was showering and sleeping. He uploaded her images and videos to porn sites, and in 2023 she was awarded nearly £100,000 for the devastating psychological impacts, as well as the costs of getting the content removed online.[3] Similarly, Love Islander and influencer Georgia Harrison, who was secretly recorded having sex, with the video shared online and on OnlyFans, secured just over £200,000 in damages (though she has not received any of the money from her perpetrator, and even if she did, most of it would be siphoned off to pay her legal costs).[4]

However, these cases are the exception. Hardly anyone knows of these options, and that's understandable, because the law can be complex, it doesn't cover every situation and basically you need a lot of money and have to find the right lawyers. But, while possible, these legal actions are hardly ever used and are not an option for most of us.

But we can change that. We can make civil law options straightforward and easily accessible. It's not difficult, and we don't have to reinvent the wheel. There are examples that we can take from within the UK in other types of dispute and in other countries that are pioneering these approaches. All we need is the determination to prioritise this issue and then take the necessary steps.

What would this look like? First, there would be new legislation creating a statutory, civil offence of image-based sexual abuse that sits alongside the criminal offences. This means that, as well as being able to report to the police if someone took or shared your intimate images, you could sue them in a civil court. The laws on harassment and stalking have similar civil and criminal provisions (though they are not used as often as they could be), and many states in the US and in Canada already have provisions like this.

In addition, that legislation would set out the kinds of court orders for which you could apply. These could be orders prohibiting offenders from distributing intimate images without consent, to delete the material, to remove it from any social media or to disable access from any online forum. Orders transferring copyright could also be made. Your perpetrator, therefore, would no longer have the images on their devices, no longer have that power and control over you. They may even be ordered to pay compensation.

Additional orders could be issued against social media companies and porn platforms to swiftly remove material on pain of significant penalties and to pay any damages where justified. We could give the courts power to block access to websites that either refuse to remove non-consensual material or do not remove flagged material in a timely manner. We could order search engines to down-rank or de-index content. There's so much that could be done to help women and girls facing this nightmare; they do not have to feel powerless and alone.

The key to the success of any such changes would be making them easily accessible, cheap and swift. We can do this: the Canadians were there before us. In British Columbia they have set up an online court process where you can complete the relevant forms online, and a judge decides the case. You don't need expensive lawyers or knowledge of complicated areas of law. What it does require is governmental commitment, determination to act, plus resourcing and effort to set it up. We already do this for all manner of other disputes, from tribunals established to regulate the pensions of war veterans, to parking charges in London, to tribunals determining access to special educational resources, so we can do it for online harms. Then of course it requires women and men affected to know about it. That needs greater awareness-raising and, ideally, support from organisations to help victims through the process. But it's all possible.

My proposal has real benefits. You decide whether to take action, what to pursue. You don't have to seek damages, you might just want the court order to remove material. You might just act against the platform that has refused to take your material down. It is true that some may see this as a burden on the victim; a benefit of the criminal justice system is that it is the responsibility of police and prosecutors to see the case through. But where it feels right, the civil law should be an option. It's about justice, accountability and empowering victims.

Using the civil law to challenge pornography is not a new idea. It was proposed decades ago by feminist icons Catharine MacKinnon and Andrea Dworkin. Back in the 1980s, they proposed a right of action against pornography producers where women could establish that they had been harmed by the pornography. What seemed radical at the time (and still is) was that they were trying to hold the producers responsible. The headlines were all about 'censorship', but that's not what it was about.

The point is that MacKinnon and Dworkin were trying new and different ways of ensuring that the producers of porn that directly harms women were held accountable. My proposals also include the possibility of seeking compensation for harms that are directly incurred and can be proven – that would mostly be financial compensation for loss of livelihood, mental health support and related costs. This would be more straightforward against a perpetrator who shares non-consensual intimate material online. But, in addition, cases can be taken against those platforms that are aware they are hosting that material but fail to do anything about it. Why should those responsible for such serious harms not be held accountable?

While my suggestions are vital and possible, getting such changes onto the agenda of law reformers is not easy. While my colleague Erika Rackley and I called for civil as well as criminal measures to tackle these harms about ten years ago, it's the criminal law that has gripped the political agenda. Indeed, without good reason, the government-commissioned review of laws on image-based abuse in 2019 specifically excluded any examination of the civil law.

But the mood music might just be changing. Over the last few years, at almost every opportunity, I've spoken in Parliament to make the case for these reforms. I'm usually asked to talk about the criminal law, but I always respond, in the same breath, to say what we also really need are civil law reforms. The heads nod, though the eyes usually glaze over. But, with the support of organisations like #NotYourPorn, the End Violence Against Women coalition and *Glamour* magazine, we are making some progress. In 2024, we launched a campaign for a comprehensive Image-Based Abuse Law that would include civil law options, as well as a few other reforms I'll talk about more later in the chapter. The Revenge Porn Helpline has similarly been asking for legal changes to block access to websites that are refusing to take down non-consensual content. Politicians and the public are beginning to realise that the criminal law alone cannot tackle this abuse, and thankfully Parliament's

Women and Equalities Committee understands this. In early 2025, they recommended a new civil law regime. This was a real moment of hope, though it was soon dashed by the government rejecting all such suggestions. The challenge continues.

FREEDOM FROM INTIMATE INTRUSIONS

Civil law reforms matter, but there are further urgent changes needed to the criminal law. Let's take the semen images I discussed in an earlier chapter, where men ejaculate over women's photos. These 'tributes', as the perpetrators call them, are all over porn sites and online communities. They're commonly alongside deepfake abuse images, with some sites providing images of well-known women and options to either deepfake or 'tribute' them. It's not unlawful to create or share such images online, which is why campaign organisations, together with Baroness Owen, recently questioned this in Parliament. I also met with the Ministry of Justice to discuss including such material within current laws, so perhaps there will be some change here soon.

The sharing of intimate images of sex workers without their consent is not covered by the current law, nor are the variety of ways in which Black and minoritised women have sexual and intimate images taken and shared without their agreement. And it's not clear whether uploading intimate images without consent to AI companions or models like ChatGPT is unlawful, partly because definitions of terms such as 'distribution' and 'the public' have not kept pace with AI developments.

Then there's the men who are creating sexualised avatars of identifiable women, without their consent, and interacting with them sexually and possibly sharing them online for others to use and abuse. Should this be allowed? I don't think so, where this is of an identifiable individual and against their will. Next, there's increasing reports of sexual abuse and harassment in the metaverse, the virtual, immersive world – the 3D iteration of the internet – we will all be occupying in the years to come, as well as the emerging ways that chatbots sexually harass users.[5] These abuses are similarly not all covered by the current law.

What I want to emphasise is that all these abusive practices are just the latest in the litany of ways technology is used to abuse women, and women's space, privacy and autonomy are invaded. Each time we uncover a new form of abuse, we search for ways to tackle it. This commonly means, first, trying to fit women's experiences into existing legal categories, usually with little success. The criminal law has not been created or interpreted with women's harms at the fore. This realisation is then followed by survivors having to speak out, campaigns being started and, finally, if we're lucky, law reform secured. However, each time, the law tends to just deal with that specific form of abuse. I've been involved in campaigns about sharing intimate images, upskirting, cyberflashing, creating and distributing deepfakes and more. Each time a very welcome new law is adopted, but very soon, the next abusive practice emerges.

The alternative is the introduction of a more general law addressing the variety of ways women are abused, and which future-proofs the law. My suggestion is a new criminal offence covering 'intimate intrusions'. Rather than accommodating women's experiences within existing criminal law categories, this new offence would take women's lived experiences as the starting point.[6] A new law could be centred on the experience of 'intimate intrusion' – an invasion, infringement of personal liberty, integrity or privacy – and cover any act of a sexual nature that would likely cause another person fear, degradation, humiliation or harm. There are examples of similar laws in many other countries, such as Sweden, which protects against violations of 'sexual integrity'.[7] The real advantage is that such a law would cover not only all existing forms of harm, but also the many ways that abuse is likely to be perpetrated in the future that we can't yet imagine.

CRIMINALISING PATRIARCHAL PORN

Next, let's reform the laws on pornography. Criminal laws against some forms of pornography, known as obscenity, have ancient roots and remain the basis of the law in the UK, as well as in the US, Canada and many other countries. Obscenity laws focus on the moral corruption of the users of porn – does the content 'deprave and corrupt' the user – rather than the harms experienced by women and society generally, meaning they are singularly unsuited to dealing with the misogyny and racism of mainstream porn. If I could reform all of the law on pornography, I would sweep away the obscenity laws and replace them with harm-based prohibitions. However, that's just not realistic. Even the recent, very comprehensive, review of porn regulation in the UK didn't touch this issue; there's just so much else to do.

My focus here then is on reforms that might just be possible. The other caveat is that I'm recommending changes to the criminal law because it provides the baseline for obligations imposed on social media and porn platforms to reduce harmful content. Their responsibilities largely relate to illegal material, and this is true in the UK with the Online Safety Act, as well as with similar laws across the European Union and elsewhere. Such a regulatory approach is not going to change any time soon. Therefore, to get Big Porn and Big Tech to do more, we need to expand the criminal law.

This starts with strengthening the law on extreme pornography. It already covers depictions of life-threatening injury, rape and serious injuries to the anus, breasts and genitals. It also covers bestiality images and necrophilia. But it does not yet include strangulation or incest.

As I write, the government has heeded calls to extend the law to cover depictions of strangulation, a reform myself and others have been recommending for a few years. If the final version of the law is comprehensive and is properly enforced by the regulator Ofcom, this will bring the online world into alignment with offline regulation, which has long prohibited depictions of strangulation. It will also represent a significant change and hopefully help reduce the normalisation of choking and strangulation in sexual life and online.

What then about incest porn? As we saw in an earlier chapter, this material is rife, reproducing the practices and justificatory narratives of child sexual abuse. That's why I would strengthen the extreme porn law to cover depictions of unlawful acts of incest and family abuse.[8] Over the last few years, I've been in Parliament a number of times making this case for reform and talking to MPs about its prevalence in Big Porn, on X, as well as Google's role in facilitating searchers for it. Many MPs were shocked and surprised by its easy availability, as they were by the fact that our current laws don't cover it. I hope this translates into their supporting reform.

Specifically, I suggest extending the extreme porn law to cover material reproducing criminal activity, meaning that it wouldn't cover just any reference to 'stepmom' or 'daddy' or similar. It's the depiction of *unlawful* sexual activity *between* family members that should be prohibited. I'm primarily targeting those videos portraying fathers, stepfathers or brothers having sex with their very young-looking daughters (and sisters). Limiting this to only unlawful activity means that representations of stepfathers having sex with their consenting 18+ stepdaughters would not be included. Such sexual activity isn't actually a criminal offence – though I think it should be in most circumstances, as these relationships have commonly involved coercion and years of grooming.

Next, we must target videos of very young-looking girls that mimic child sexual abuse, even though the actors are aged eighteen or over. You'll recall that so often it is not just that the girls look young, but we are encouraged to think this by all the childhood surroundings, the bedding, the clothes, the toys and the language used. While this material is prohibited offline, such regulations are largely pointless in the age of online Big Porn.

Surprisingly, these images do not fall within current laws on child sexual abuse material. English law only includes images of children, defined as those under eighteen. The law is stronger in other countries, such as Ireland, where the law extends to *depictions* of a child. This is the same in a number of Australian states and New Zealand, where laws refer to images that 'appear to be' or are 'implied to be' of children. Canadian law goes one step further, and also prohibits any material, written or visual, that 'advocates' sexual activity with a child.

Now, there will always be images that are borderline. When does the video *appear to be* a child? When is something advocacy?

But we need a law to tackle the images that are so clearly intended to look like young girls. This content legitimises gaining sexual gratification from child sexual abuse; it validates it. The Canadian provision would equally target the online communities that brazenly talk of their own sexual activity with young girls, particularly stepdaughters, encouraging it (even if what they are saying is not true) and applauding the material being displayed – that's advocacy for child sexual abuse.

The need for action is ever more pressing since the advent of AI. As things stand, if AI is used to create an image of sexual activity where the 'impression conveyed' is of a child, such as a girl looking around 13–14 years, it is classed as unlawful child sexual abuse material. You can be convicted of creating, sharing or possessing it, and imprisoned for up to ten years. But an identical video made with an 18+ actor, even though they look so very young, is lawful. We are in the bizarre situation of prohibiting the AI image because we recognise that such material promotes, encourages and legitimises child sexual abuse, but not the one with an actor over eighteen, though this has the same impact and effect. The intention is the same, the harm is the same and the law should be the same.

CONTROLLING PLATFORMS

While changes to criminal and civil laws are vital, the reality is that, if we are going to reduce the harms of mainstream porn, it is Big Tech and Big Porn that must be made to act. We are beginning to see greater regulation of internet platforms through legislation in the UK, such as the Online Safety Act, and the European

Union has similar laws in place. But there is almost no appetite for regulation in the US, where so many of the major platforms are based. Also, while some of these laws are moving in the right direction, it remains to be seen whether they actually will be enforced. The omens are not good. The largest tech platforms have all rowed back from commitments to trust and safety at the behest of Donald Trump.

I participated in the inter-governmental summit on AI in Paris in February 2025, attended by heads of government, where the idealism of AI and the need to encourage innovation at all costs dominated debate. The first such summit had been convened by the UK in 2023, and was called the AI *safety* summit. By 2025, safety had been erased from the lexicon, and we were now at an *action* summit, though unfortunately that did not mean action to reduce harms. It was clear to me that we had learned nothing from the havoc wreaked by the free-for-all of social media; it was all full speed ahead, worry about failures and harms later. We seemed to have collectively forgotten that allowing tech platforms to self-regulate and prioritise profit results in significant and devastating harms for so many, and leaves our democratic institutions at the mercy of algorithms. In the context of porn, the anything goes mentality has led to the world of patriarchal porn. Internet idealism has been resurrected as AI idealism.

It is in this political context that we have to consider how to control Big Porn and Big Tech. So I can tell you what the law is and what regulators could be doing, but whether any steps are actually taken to curb the harms of porn remains to be seen. The UK's Online Safety Act 2023 has the laudable aim of creating safer online environments, and tries to do this by imposing duties on platforms to protect users from harmful content. The good thing is that this is supposed to be done at the systems level. This means that, rather than just being a legal regime taking down harmful material, the aim is to stop it being there in the first place, emphasising safety by design. Platforms are supposed to review policies and processes, such as their algorithms and their promotion of harmful content, as well as policies on the ease of uploading content and financial incentives for doing so.

So far so good. As ever though, the reality is not as good as the rhetoric, and there are serious questions about whether much will change. Realistically, the prospects were never good. The original 262-page draft of the Online Safety Bill did not mention women and girls once, despite it being known that women are disproportionately subject to online abuse, particularly Black and racially minoritised women. In response, a large coalition of specialist organisations and experts on violence against women – me included – worked tirelessly to get some specific requirements into the Act. It was quite some battle – remarkable really that there was such resistance – and we did manage to get the legislation changed. However, all we got was that the regulator Ofcom must produce best practice guidance for platforms on tackling online violence against women and girls. It's very good *guidance*, but may make little difference, especially in the current climate, as it's not legally enforceable.

A similarly determined campaign was required to strengthen the rules on Big Porn. While requirements to reduce children's access were eventually included, the government resisted all moves to harmonise the offline and online regulation of pornography (which would have meant a considerable reduction in the prevalence of harmful porn online). As a compromise, it set up a review of all pornography regulation, kicking any real change into the long grass. Then, even once the porn review had reported, the new government sat on it for a long time. So far, the government has committed to extending the extreme porn law to cover strangulation, but we await any change to regulation and action against the platforms.

This reluctance to take bold action regarding either pornography or violence against women and girls is reflected in how the legislation is being put into practice by the regulator Ofcom. It has the role of interpreting the legislation, providing the guidance for Big Tech and Big Porn and then enforcing the law. Unfortunately, Ofcom's approach has been hugely disappointing, as made clear by many charities working to reduce harms against women and children. The hope that the legislation would require a step change in how Big Tech operated rapidly fizzled out, replaced by despair and deep disappointment. The lobbying of Big Tech and Big Porn was, as ever, highly effective, with many instances of guidance being watered down (even further) at their behest. Then, any hope for a change in approach was firmly squashed by the political headwinds from the US and the UK government prioritising corporate investment and 'innovation' at the expense of safety and reduction in harms.

Nonetheless, let's dive into some of the specifics to see what might still be possible. First, we need to address the issue of age-assurance, designed to reduce children's easy access to online pornography. My key point with age-assurance laws is that, while worthy, they are too often a distraction from the main problem, which is the *content* of Big Porn. Frankly, we would not be so concerned about children accessing porn were it not for the horrific nature of the content on mainstream platforms. Imagine if all the energy and money that has gone into age-assurance had been spent transforming the content of porn; we would not need age-assurance laws, and I would not have had to write this book.

However, we are where we are, and age-assurance laws are being introduced around the world. Don't get me wrong, seeing as the content of Big Porn is unlikely to change much in the immediate future, we do need to do something to reduce young children's easy access. This is particularly urgent for the youngest who stumble across material, often leaving them destabilised and upset. It's necessary so that we can reduce the impact of Big Porn on the behaviours, attitudes and developing brains of teenagers. At the same time, we must be alive to the risk of pushing people to smaller platforms that are even more immune from regulation.

When we examine the specifics of how age-assurance might work, we need to see through the propaganda of Big Porn. As I write, age-assurance laws are coming into force in the UK, and Pornhub is on a PR offensive. They're trying to win over the public by playing on people's ignorance by repeatedly stating that there are huge privacy concerns around giving your personal data to porn platforms. But this is not what these laws require! Age-assurance is secured via third party providers with strong privacy protections. This means that, while pornography sites are required to reduce underage access, they need not receive or store any personally identifiable information. However, the irony must not be lost that Pornhub is trying to stoke fears over privacy violations when it is relentlessly harvesting and selling the data of its users.

The porn and social media platforms are also trying to convince us that what they call 'device-level' age restrictions should be introduced instead, meaning that, when you buy a phone, for example, you state whether it will be used by an adult or a child. Of course they are pushing this idea (even though it's not yet clear how this would technically work) because it would mean that they would not have to change any of their practices and could keep making a profit while putting the onus on users. The reality is that this idea would be pointless because of the ease of getting around any such initial restriction, and the sharing of devices. Nothing would change, which is what they want.

Let's focus then on actually regulating the content. Technically, the online safety law requires the largest porn platforms, such as Pornhub, XVideos and XHamster, to take preventative action to ensure users don't encounter illegal material and, if they do find such material, it should be swiftly removed. Illegal content includes extreme pornography such as rape porn and acts depicting life-threatening or serious injury. In addition, it includes image-based abuse material, such as sexually explicit deepfakes, and these rules similarly apply to social media companies including X, which we know is awash with porn and non-consensual material.

What does this all mean in practice? It means there should no longer be rape porn on the mainstream platforms, and that includes all the sleep, stealthing and force material. But it's still all there. Is the regulator going to properly enforce this law? I fear not, though I hope I am wrong. If the law on extreme porn is expanded to include strangulation, and possibly incest, then that material too would also need to be removed. That would be a lot of content to be taken down. That of course is the whole point. But for such changes to have any real meaning, the regulator must act.

What about Google? The Online Safety Act applies to search engines. They are meant to run their service in ways to reduce the risk of individuals coming across illegal material. While search services cannot remove content, their power lies in down-ranking and/or de-indexing content. What are we going to expect of them? There are some obvious changes, such as blocking 'asleep porn' as well as 'sleep porn'; maybe don't allow the search for 'stealthing porn'; down-rank searches for sexually explicit deepfakes without having to wait for victims to report sites. But even such changes would be largely performative.

And then there's X. Is it going to be made to remove the rape, incest and other illegal material online? Again, don't listen to any complaints about over-burdening business (notwithstanding that they have plenty of resources anyway). Simple word searches would remove so much of this material. Also, watch out for when they remove far more content than they need to, making claims of forced censorship. That's their playbook: saying they've done what is required and it's too much, all to try to convince us that the law goes 'too far'. It doesn't.

If we started on this regulatory journey, the content of Big Porn would change. If we started removing unlawful material from porn platforms and reduced access via search engines to rape porn or similar websites, we might begin to shift attitudes away from thinking force and exploitation is a normal part of sexual arousal. The police officer and the jury member might associate the evidence they are being given not with the normal, everyday porn they watch online, but with unlawful acts of sexual violence. Young women might not be faced quite so often with men trying to strangle them during sex without even discussing it, thinking that's what they want or expect. It might not even enter the heads of teenage boys to take videos up the skirts of their women teachers, as they've not been groomed to think that it's a worthwhile, funny and acceptable genre online. Websites might swiftly respond to reports of unlawful material being uploaded, or even require written consent of all those in videos before uploading.

Slowly but surely, the content would change, our perceptions and norms would change. For the better. Remember, it hasn't always been this way, and it doesn't have to be this way forever after.

TAKING THE FIGHT TO BIG TECH AND BIG PORN

To take the challenge to Big Porn and Big Tech, we need a new regulator for online harms and pornography with additional new powers. This might sound techy or bureaucratic, but it could make a huge difference. My suggestion is an Online Safety Commission or Commissioner – an agile, expert, empowered, proactive regulator that can prioritise pornography regulation and take direct steps to reduce harms. The Commission could be a public voice to champion reform, a leading player on the world stage, known for its action. It could have powers to act directly against recalcitrant websites and porn platforms, issue orders to get material taken down within specified time limits and support individual complaints. It could introduce mandatory consent requirements regarding all participants in pornographic material online. It could issue binding rules for porn platforms and social media on how fast and effective procedures must be in place for receiving reports and actioning them. It could play a key role in educating the public, awareness campaigns, training activities and guidance for schools. It could require deterrent messaging on porn websites, to divert users away from unlawful material. It could force search engines to down-rank harmful material in ways far more effective than the current rhetoric. It could provide specialist support, information and advocacy to victims of abuse. It could do so many things to disrupt patriarchal porn and to alter the current climate in which it thrives.

The reality is that the current UK regulator, Ofcom, is too general; its remit covers a vast range of industries, meaning it cannot prioritise pornography and online abuse. It has shown in its interpretation and implementation of the Online Safety Act that it is more concerned with the 'costs' and perceived burdens on tech companies, with far less consideration of the cost of online harms and abuse to women, girls and wider society. It privileges the speech rights of platforms and users/abusers over victims of online abuse.[9]

My suggestion isn't pie in the sky. There are regulators around the world that have many of these powers, though admittedly not one that has them all. But we could be pioneers. And there are examples of robust regulators close to home. Take advertising. The UK's Advertising Standards Authority has power to ban sexist adverts, and it uses its powers. Recently, it acted against an online game that advertised 'roleplay with AI stepmom'. It featured a text chat sent by 'Stepmom' saying, 'Your dad is away for a while … What are you going to do?' The reply stated, 'I guess you can show me something in your room [winking face emoji]'. There was also a suggestion of a 'student' AI with an image of a young girl in school uniform.[10] They banned it for promoting stepfamily sexual activity and sexualising an under-eighteen. It is great that the Advertising Standards Authority makes these rulings. But what is incredible is that we have that system alongside the total absence of regulation of far more extreme material in mainstream porn that is viewed by millions every minute of every day. Why is this prohibited in adverts but not porn?

MORE RIGHTS, FEWER RISKS IN THE PORN INDUSTRY

Then there's regulation of the porn industry itself. It's difficult to be definitive about the exploitative nature of the industry, as it's obviously vast, global and highly fragmented, and so we cannot speak in monolithic terms. Nonetheless, we know that many performers, especially young women, enter the industry under desperate conditions, whether they be financial, lack of other opportunities, false inducements or the influence of coercive partners and recruiters.[11] The recent independent review of pornography in the UK – the Bertin Review – found that, while the true extent of trafficking and exploitation in the industry is unknown, when women do come forward their experiences are often harrowing.[12] The review further reported that safety protocols across the pornography industry are 'inconsistent', meaning that content is produced where creators have been coerced into performing, and where age-checks have not been sufficient. It recommended, therefore, new requirements for written and documented proof of consent and age verification.

We know that many performers in the industry, even if not all, are vulnerable due to experiences of poverty, prior victimisation and other disadvantages, including addiction and mental ill-health.[13] And the boundaries between lawful activities and trafficking have become more difficult to determine in recent years, due to the rapidly changing nature of the industry, particularly the shift away from production companies to online performances, camming [webcam performers] and the growth of sites such as OnlyFans.[14]

Even when not trafficked, performers may face exploitative contracts, unsafe working conditions and pressure to consent to acts to which they did not initially agree. Power imbalances between producers and performers leave many with little ability to negotiate, and some describe practices amounting to intimidation or manipulation rather than genuine consent. While some people within the industry speak positively about their experiences, these perspectives, however valid, cannot erase the structural vulnerabilities that shape the entry and participation of so many others.

For these reasons, the Bertin Review set out a package of measures to improve conditions in the industry, including greater rights for performers to withdraw consent to the distribution of their porn content. Pornography is recorded, distributed and made permanently accessible to audiences across the world, and it's this permanence that makes the right to withdraw consent particularly important. A performer may initially agree to a scene or video but later come to understand the personal, professional or psychological consequences differently, deciding, for example, that having their image available indefinitely exposes them to stigma and harassment, and may well limit their future work opportunities. Reforms that enable performers to revoke consent and have their material removed would acknowledge the unique and enduring risks they face. Companies hosting pornographic content, therefore, would need to have clear and standardised processes to ensure that performers and creators can withdraw consent and have content removed online promptly.

One response to such a proposal is that there would not be the same risks of abuse and stigma if working in the industry was not shrouded in such shame and controversy. And that's true. However, while we are where we are, and the reality and public perception of the industry is unlikely to change in the near future, performers should be granted rights to withdraw consent.

The Bertin Review offered a range of recommendations to make the industry more transparent in its activities and provide information to the public about the operation of platforms and companies, enabling us all to make more informed choices about our viewing. An accreditation scheme was set out that would inform the public about which companies and platforms are compliant with the law and actively tackling unlawful content online. The ideal is that this would lead to more traffic to those platforms, rather than others not accredited; it would also enable banks, payment providers and other associated businesses to make more ethical and informed choices.

CREATING PORN WITHOUT PATRIARCHY

At the same time as trying to restrict the morass of harmful porn, and better control the industry, we need to look at the possibility of pursuing sexual liberty and sexual representation on our own and different terms. This means asking, what would porn without patriarchy actually look like?

A common mantra when debating porn regulation is that the 'answer to bad porn isn't no porn. It's better porn.'[15] This 'better porn' is commonly labelled ethical, feminist or indie porn. There are of course many different interpretations of what constitutes 'feminist' porn and, as a label, it's certainly been co-opted to rebrand what is actually problematic porn. But, at its best, feminist porn arises from a political vision, a social movement challenging mainstream racist, sexist, heteronormative and ablest portrayals of sexual activity.[16] So feminist porn producers and actors will talk about portraying consent, women's pleasure, about people of different gender identities, races, body types or abilities that are not fetishised or stereotyped. It also embraces ethical values encompassing fair pay and safe, consensual working conditions for actors and producers. It's about a broader vision of gender equality and social justice, liberating women and men.

Recently, the term 'indie porn' has become more common than 'feminist', with writer and performer Zahra Stardust talking about how indie porn is imagining different ways for governments, companies and all of us as individuals to value desire and pleasure. The focus is on health, well-being, rights and diversity of performers and producers, as well as collaborative decision-making, transparency, sharing of profits, all challenging the capitalist practices of conventional, commercial pornography. Stardust speaks of nothing less than the potential of indie porn to change and liberate our relationships not only with sex but also with media, society and capitalism.[17]

These genres of porn are part of a social movement with broad aims, and their method of persuasion to try to transform society is through sexual media and representations. So while there is a spectrum of what might be labelled as 'feminist' or 'indie' porn, it includes performance artists embracing the culture, values and political outlook of feminism. Ingrid Ryberg, a feminist porn filmmaker and artist, talks about how feminist porn, both aesthetically and politically, draws on feminist political activism around women's rights to sexual self-determination and bodily autonomy. Feminist porn, she says, is about the 'practice of imagining alternatives and a safe space for sexual empowerment'.[18]

Feminist porn producers are saying, let us harness pornography's persuasive force to shape attitudes and behaviours and change the message to a more egalitarian vision of gender and sexuality.[19] If patriarchal porn functions as propaganda spreading misogynistic and racist sexual scripts, then feminist pornography is a significant, if not unique, method of challenge and change. And this is likely to be far more effective than, say, a public campaign about attitudes or sex education, as it utilises the strength of associations with pleasure and orgasm.[20]

You can probably see the obvious stumbling block. How would we ever get the consumers of mainstream porn to switch to feminist porn? If mainstream porn inculcates attitudes that are patriarchal, why would they start, voluntarily, watching feminist porn? It's not like we could use public funds to mandate watching feminist porn, and a lot of it, to ensure that the repeated egalitarian messaging is taken on board.[21]

Nonetheless, there is some appetite for porn without patriarchy, for something more authentic, less abusive, more real, more imaginative, more fulfilling, more ethically satisfying. Feminist porn producer Erika Lust calls for us to be more 'mindful' in our search for erotic content. But it is hard to find. Many women talk about wanting to find something else, but it's just too difficult.[22] Partly this is because there is so little of it out there; it truly is a drop in the ocean, though there are articles in mainstream magazines trying to raise these issues.[23] There are financial and structural issues that could address this, though, such as enabling greater investment in ethical and feminist porn from mainstream banking, as powerfully put forward by Cindy Gallop, the creator of the #MakeLoveNotPorn website, who has been promoting authentic porn for many years.[24] The UK independent review of pornography further recommended changes to end the 'financial discrimination' against many who work in the porn sector, which, if accompanied by the proposed accreditation scheme, could mean greater investment and support in smaller, ethical companies.

Feminist and indie porn is providing a challenge to the dominance of mainstream porn. However, while some say that, rather than regulating the mainstream, we just have to keep on making more and more and better and better feminist porn, we need to do both. I can't see how feminist and indie porn, on their own, without a change in either the content or business model of mainstream porn, can make much of an impact. Similarly, we may enjoy indie films, but they're not going to change how Hollywood produces and sells its movies. Robust regulation is vital to free us from patriarchal porn, so that our lives may flourish and in doing so enable more feminist porn.

RECLAIMING SEX EDUCATION FROM BIG PORN

Reforming the porn industry and supporting indie, feminist alternatives are vital steps, but on their own they are not enough. And while my central focus has been on strengthening regulation and law reform providing the foundation for lasting change, we must transform how young people are educated about sex, consent and pornography. Right now, we've handed sex education over to Big Porn. Any teaching in schools is patchy and inconsistent, with young people often describing it as irrelevant or useless. It's too often delivered by teachers without the training or expertise to deal with the subject properly. This is not a marginal issue: it shapes how new generations understand intimacy, respect and relationships, and how they might navigate the online world. But if sex and relationships education is to meet that challenge, it must be properly funded, expert-led and available to all.[25]

I'm certainly not the first to make such a call; indeed it's such a common suggestion that it's sometimes dismissed as little more than a mantra. But the truth is, if we got this right, the impact could be transformative. Comprehensive, expert education could equip young people to navigate an online world saturated with pornography and help them to understand consent – but also joy and pleasure. Ethical conduct – it can give them tools to question harmful messages about sex and gender. Some organisations already show what is possible: Beyond Equality, for instance, runs powerful programmes with boys and young men that open up conversations about masculinity, relationships and responsibility.[26] Expanding and sustaining this kind of work could change not just individual lives but the wider culture in which patriarchal pornography currently thrives.

TURNING THE TIDE

In the early days of the internet, there was a powerful idealism about how it was going to democratise the world, give a voice to everyone, enable connections, unleash our imagination. Porn was included in this vision, supposedly ushering in an era where we could view any porn we wanted, a smorgasbord of sexual appetites and tastes to suit every desire that would liberalise sex, release the marginalised and open new avenues of exploration, fantasy and arousal. Neither of these visions have materialised and, in fact, everything we know about Big Tech and Big Porn is that it has destructive tendencies overpowering any positive gains.

There were a brief few years when it was acknowledged that Big Tech was in fact a force for harm, rather than for good, and that self-regulation had failed. We saw the takedown of millions of videos from Pornhub; we heard the details of whistleblowers from Facebook; and we saw the introduction of the Online Safety Act and its equivalent in the European Union. Note that this was the time of #MeToo, when misogyny and sexual violence were being challenged on a global scale.

Now, however, we are feeling the backlash. Governments and regulators are bowing down to Big Tech and Big Porn, which seem more powerful than ever before, not least due to the AI revolution. The backlash has the same hyper-masculine flavour that currently dominates politics and social media. It's leading to the removal of trust and safety staff and programmes, as well as an AI free-for-all. It's anti-equality, with the male influencers and tech bros unashamedly propagating ideas of masculine dominance.

We have got a fight on our hands to shift the debate back towards the regulation of Big Tech and in particular curtailing Big Porn. Porn must be regulated to ensure that women and girls can live free from violence and abuse, as well as having the freedom and liberty to choose their own paths. Without effective regulation, platforms prioritise engagement and profit over safety, allowing harmful content to flourish. To reiterate, regulation is not about limiting expression – it is in fact about enabling the free expression of women and girls, ensuring that women and girls are not pushed offline through fear and intimidation. Regulation is vital in order to enable us to live the lives we choose. While these arguments may run counter to prevailing sentiment, we must keep making them in the hope that one day the tide will turn.

Conclusion: Reclaiming Sexual Freedom and Desire

Towards the end of writing this book, I stumbled upon a video on X that was simply titled 'public toilet'. The woman, quite literally, has a toilet seat placed over her head. She's kneeling on the ground and various men are urinating directly into her mouth and all over her head and body. They urinate and ejaculate directly into her eyes; she struggles to keep them wide open. She smiles wanly to the camera every now and then to convince us that she's OK. Her head is forcefully held and hit while gagging on a penis. After two minutes of this (which feels like a very long time), her face is forced onto the floor and held there by a man's foot, her arms held behind her back by another, and she is made to lick urine off the floor.

'Public toilet' is a quintessential example of patriarchal porn, a woman's humiliation being eroticised. It is revelling in women's degradation and powerlessness. Not only sexualising her subordination, but showing us she enjoys it. The acquiescence, her feeble smile to the camera, makes this worse than if she were obviously being coerced: it symbolises the true success of patriarchal values. She accepts and wants to be oppressed, humiliated, degraded, treated like a toilet.

This video is not currently unlawful. It's true that this sort of content would once have been deemed obscene, but no longer, at least not in any legal sense, as it's not depicting illegal activities. Nor is it extreme porn. It's possible, though unlikely, that it might be prohibited offline but, in any event, offline regulation has little relevance to the porn being viewed online today.

In any event, it's never likely to be unlawful, and probably never should be. This is the real challenge with this sort of porn: it's abusive and misogynistic, but there are limits to the law. Even if we implemented all my suggestions from the last chapter, 'public toilet' could still be lawfully produced, distributed and viewed, perhaps by millions.

PATRIARCHAL PORN LOATHES WOMEN

Patriarchal porn is not about sex; instead it uses sex as a method by which to showcase and entrench misogyny. We see this most clearly in videos such as 'public toilet'. That video is not just about urolagnia, the sexual paraphilia of gaining sexual gratification from urination. There are lots of urination videos in mainstream porn, including women peeing on men. But many, such as 'public toilet', involving men urinating on women, are not about sexual arousal but humiliation and oppression. The men may have erections and may ejaculate, but it is not a sense of sexual satisfaction that is being conveyed. It's power: consolidated, maintained, enforced.

This is emblematic of much lawful mainstream porn, such as the multiple variations on the theme of 'dumb black bitch' or 'stupid blonde cunt', encouraging women to be seen as so unworthy that anything can be done to or said about them. Dehumanised. It's further evident in the more obviously abusive content, such as the video 'scared crying teen gets pounded', discussed earlier. That young girl was being raped, strangled, gagged and slapped, all in the name of sexual arousal, though that really didn't seem to be what it was about. As well as the obvious physical abuse, there was an underlying air of cruelty, as if her very existence was aggravating and provoking him, that she was still there, putting up with it, making him furious.

Porn is full of loathing for women and girls. It's ostensibly about sexual arousal, sexual pleasure, but it embodies hate, anger, aggression and humiliation. So many men in these porn videos seem to detest women and girls. There are, of course, other types of material on these websites and across social media that might be more conventionally understood as basic porn for sexual arousal. But my point is about the overall ethos and effect of the genre. It's also not only about specific physical acts. Some specialist BDSM material is stylised, carefully crafted, clearly physically demanding and harmful, but without this sense of disgust and loathing. To emphasise, though, that is not the material abundant in Big Porn.

This is where we also need to remind ourselves that men, like women, can be motivated to pursue sex for non-sexual reasons. They may also feel the need to assert their masculinity, motivated by the link between ejaculation, erection and power.[1] It's not that women have reasons and incentives for sex – comfort, building a relationship, preventing violence – and men only desire, yet we rarely consider men's non-sexual motivations. We treat male arousal as inherently biological, rather than seeing it as produced by, and then sanctioned by, society. This echoes the fact that it's little recognised that sexual violence is not only about sexual gratification, but far more about exerting power, humiliation, revenge, punishment, relieving boredom and simply because it's possible.

These are the stimuli we see in so much porn. Not only are we watching the depiction of these differing motives, of power, punishment and more, but we are seeing them being sustained through their repetition, their ease of availability, and through the community engagement and participation they inspire by being on large platforms with extensive user activity. In time, this reshapes the basis for desire, as sexual arousal develops in a social context. Patriarchal porn plays a central role in the construction of this form of masculinity, by encouraging exertions of power in a world where some men have little power and where they are encouraged to think it is women who have taken their power.

Some of this material on X is so obvious you'd think it was a parody (it isn't). One video is headlined 'nothing is hotter than misogynistic porn that promotes abusing women'. This accompanies a video of a woman being raped, slapped and strangled by multiple men as she screams. You also can easily find porn content labelled 'anti-feminism'. Remember the comment that accompanies the video 'daddy forces stepdaughter': 'sometimes you just gotta #MeToo the bitch'.[2]

These are the sentiments we see reproduced every day online by male influencers of the Andrew Tate brand. His description of sexual acts, of what men should be doing, of women's role, is absolutely about exerting power and control, domination. There is no hiding from it, nor from the fact that the male influencers dominate the social media of younger men, and that millions are engaging with Big Porn.

PORN SILENCES WOMEN (AND SOME MEN)

It is this loathing that makes mainstream porn so impactful. It affects every area of our social, cultural and political worlds because of its power and authority. This porn is the ideological and cultural scaffolding of inequality in general: power and control over women, maintaining our subordination, restricting our liberty, enforcing hierarchies of gender, race, ethnicity and ability. This is why it is vital to understand this pornography not as just *depicting* patriarchy, but producing it, sustaining it and enforcing it. It's not just a representation, but designs our subordination, through violence and abuse, making it real.

One of the main ways this porn secures its ambition is by silencing women (and some men).[3] I've talked about this most directly in relation to deepfake sexual abuse, where women, particularly those in the public eye, are targeted with the aim of pushing them out of public life, to make them self-censor and think twice about what they are doing and saying. However, this silencing is far more extensive and insidious, affecting us all.[4]

The sexual scripts make it harder for women and girls to protest against unwanted sex, and harder for men to hear our protests or to voice their own desires. They make it harder for women to share their experience of abuse, to be believed; harder for women, men, juries, police officers, the public to hear their reports and stories of harm. They make it harder for us to express our sexual desires, to even know our sexual desires; harder for our wants to be understood, respected. They make it harder for us to be seen, to be heard, to be taken seriously. They make it harder for us to be more than a fuckable, usable, disposable body. We scream in porn, but no one notices, or if they do, they think that's an acceptable part of the excitement. We scream in real life, and few hear or care, inured to harm, inequality, abuse, humiliation and oppression.

If porn is silencing women, that means that our rights to free speech are being infringed. But while laws protecting freedom of expression do apply, they are not applied in the service of the rights of women and girls. As I discussed earlier, debates are characterised as a fight between (men's) rights to pornography and censorship. This dominant framing continues, rather than us recognising that it is in fact Big Porn and Big Tech that are controlling what we read and how we speak, that free speech is restricted in all manner of ways and for good reasons, such as prohibitions on shouting 'fire' in crowded rooms or 'kill' to an attack dog.

The American legal scholar Mary Ann Franks sets this out so well, reminding us that free speech rights are always available to defend men's misogynistic expression and sexual exploitation, such as when the first non-consensual nudes of Marilyn Monroe were published in the launch edition of *Playboy*.[5] Progress for women is often tolerated, but only insofar as it does not disturb what is seen as men's entitlements. When women's interests diverge from those of men, the latter's rights are reasserted to ensure they take precedence. This becomes especially clear in relation to pornography, where women's pursuit of sexual freedom and autonomy is framed as directly clashing with men's supposed entitlement to porn.

What becomes clear is that challenging mainstream porn will never be easy and the methods of resistance will be varied and extensive. We will need to endure the rage of patriarchy feeling threatened. This itself is nothing new. Historian Mary Beard has reminded us that, 'when it comes to silencing women, Western culture has had thousands of years of practice'.[6]

THE END OF PATRIARCHY

This book has exposed how porn has changed, how it's become more extreme, and how mainstream porn is best understood as patriarchal due to the values it embodies and preaches. I've argued that our debates over how to regulate mainstream porn must change, to reflect the algorithmic business model of Big Tech and Big Porn.

Patriarchal porn sexualises women's inferior status, women's inequality and women's fear. It eroticises masculine superiority and authority. It sexualises force. It sexualises sexism and racism. We must continue to fight for nothing less than an end to patriarchy, and that will only come when we fight back against the porn that sustains it.

Acknowledgements

Writing this book has been a serious challenge. Delving into the abyss online has induced deep despair on many occasions, despite me having worked in this field for decades. The combination of the cruel, misogynistic nature of the content, dripping with the loathing of women, with the reality that it's being watched by millions, and that our political masters care little, is really tough to understand and process. In addition, this is not a classic academic text, with its necessarily detached style, even though as feminist scholars we write in different ways, more open, accessible, acknowledging our position and perspectives. Righteous anger has infused every sentence in this book, an exhausting process. In writing this book, at this stage of my career, I've been reflecting on the past decades and the shifting landscape of pornography and violence against women and girls, and let us just say, it's been a disheartening process.

Suffice to say, therefore, the combination of all these factors has led me to rely heavily on others during the writing process. I owe a considerable debt of gratitude to so many who have shaped my ideas over the years, and to those who have lived with 'the book' shadowing so many conversations.

My thinking on pornography has been shaped by close working with so many truly impressive colleagues. Fiona Vera-Gray is an intellectual powerhouse, and I've benefited from our collaboration over many years, from the activism of the 'ban rape porn' campaign ten years ago, to our porn content analysis that features in many chapters, and to more recent work on policing sexual violence. Fiona has offered insightful comments and suggestions on the whole book. It was also Fiona who I turned to when feeling deep despair about the porn world we are living in, and when I was struggling to carry on in the face of overwhelming misogyny. She helped me offload and then find the will to carry on; I am eternally grateful.

My step into pornography research began with colleagues Nicole Westmarland and Erika Rackley at Durham University about twenty years ago, when we responded to the fiery public debate on extreme porn by bringing into debate many diverse voices. That was the first of many controversies to manage in this field, and Nicole has been a constant source of support and insight over decades working together. I learn so much from her, not only intellectually, but also through her academic practice. She truly embodies feminist values of care, responsibility and support, so often working behind the scenes in ways that are rarely recognised. Erika and I worked together to develop many ideas that are now part of mainstream thinking, particularly our work on image-based sexual abuse, as well as how we shaped debates on the cultural harms of extreme pornography. Her intellectual strength is immense. She is generous of spirit and full of grace.

Academic work can be isolating, especially work that goes against the grain of prevailing academic and institutional priorities. I've benefited hugely therefore from an extensive network of colleagues who motivate and support each other. My ideas have been shaped through valuable conversations with Joanne Conaghan, Sharon Cowan, Fiona de Londras, Nicola Henry, Kelly

Johnson, Liz Kelly, Vanessa Munro and Aoife O'Donoghue. Nicola Gavey has been a particular support in writing about pornography, sharing my sense of despair, the nuances of the debates, and encouraging me after speaking at events that left me shaking with despair and rage: I was not alone.

My work also builds on the research of so many impressive feminist legal scholars who I've had the honour of knowing over many years and whose scholarship is genuinely inspiring, including Janine Benedet, Karen Boyle, Michelle Burman, Danielle Keats Citron, Mary Ann Franks, Lise Gotell, Isabel Grant and Catharine MacKinnon. There are many others I never knew and don't know but whose work continues to inspire, including Andrea Dworkin (whose epitaph should be 'I told you so'), Judith Lewis Herman's groundbreaking work on incest that lit the fire under my incest porn chapter (as well as her work on justice), and Carol Gilligan's original work on ethics of care and more recent writing on patriarchy. Elaine Craig's recent book on mainstream pornography is powerful and has helped shape and bolster many of my arguments. I'm grateful to my co-authors and collaborators across many projects, including Ulrika Andersson, Hannah Bows, Katrin Hohl, Rosemary Hunter, Ruth Friskney, Carlotta Rigotti, Olivia Smith, Rüya Tuna Toparlak and Linnea Wegerstad. Thank you to Sonia Harris-Short for sharing the challenges of navigating professional life, particularly when trying to shift institutions towards more egalitarian approaches to work, life and change.

This book is a weaving of academic research, policy engagement and advocacy. I am indebted to the many survivors who have trusted me with their stories so that their experiences might help others. You have shaped my thinking, from sexual violence survivors talking about their perceptions of justice to women who

ACKNOWLEDGEMENTS

have experienced all forms of image-based sexual abuse. I am honoured to have walked the path with Sally Rees, the courageous school teacher from Northern Ireland who refused to tolerate her experience of upskirting by a pupil being swept under the carpet. I have been pleased to work with her and colleagues during the long legal battle, ultimately changing how the law was interpreted, as well as securing legislative change. She has helped me see what is possible, as well as what needs to change. Most recently, it's been a privilege to know Jodie, whose experiences of online harassment and deepfake sexual abuse, and whose determination to use her experience for the benefit of others, has genuinely inspired me and helped me carry on.

Change is only possible through working closely with organisations on the front line, who are the first to identify new trends in abuse through their work with survivors, and who mobilise civil society to insist on reform. I would like to thank Holly Dustin and Sarah Green for their work and collaboration at the End Violence Against Women coalition, and that first 'ban rape porn' campaign that has since shaped many law reforms efforts. More recently, Andrea Noble, Rebecca Hitchin, Lily O'Farrell and Sinead Geoghegan from EVAW have all inspired me with their insights and reflective approach to policy engagement. I've particularly learned so much from Sophie Mortimer of the Revenge Porn Helpline and Sandy Brindley at Rape Crisis Scotland. Lucy Morgan from *Glamour*, Elena Michael of #NotYourPorn and Sophie Compton, who founded #MyImageMyChoice, have been inspiring collaborators on the path towards change. Lorna Woods and Maeve Walsh have been stalwarts of the online safety campaigns, providing valuable advice and guidance to myself and so many. Laura Bates blazed the trail of saying the unsayable and encouraged me in my goal of sharing the nature of the patriarchal porn available online. It's also an international battle, and I've particularly benefited from sharing many platforms with Silvia Semenzin and Shanley McLaren, learning from them about priorities, 'pleasure activism' and never giving up.

I've worked with politicians of all the major political parties to try to strengthen the law. There are determined women (and some men) from across the political spectrum willing to challenge both conventional thinking and their own political parties. Cross-party work can be challenging, requiring compromise. I've always felt that so often we share common goals and that working together, and compromising, brings greater benefits.

I would like to extend my considerable thanks to Vicky Butterby, whose research assistance throughout this project, and help finalising the text, has been invaluable. Her comments and reassurance have been very welcome. In addition, Alishya Dhir provided valuable research assistance, and I'm particularly grateful to her and Sukhwant Dhaliwal for their insights on the issues relating to Black and minoritised women and girls in particular.

My professional life has been based mostly at Durham University, and I'm grateful to many colleagues over the years for their support of my work, including most recently Volker Röben, the Dean of the Law School.

This book came about through the vision of my editor, Cecilia Stein, who wanted to shine a light on the dark side of mainstream pornography, and my agent Caroline Hardman, who made this possible. I am grateful for their vision and for allowing me to take on this mantle.

I want to share my profound gratitude for the wisdom and support of Kay Young, my executive coach of many years, who

ACKNOWLEDGEMENTS

has helped me shape my professional life and stick to my path – indeed to find my path. She's also been constant in her support of this project, recognising the toll it has taken, at the same time as understanding its centrality to how I see my role in the world. She understood my sense that I had to write this book, even though that probably wasn't the best idea in view of all my other commitments. I deliberately stepped into the 'hole in the sidewalk'. But I only had awareness of what I was doing thanks to Kay. I also have Susie, always there, thank you from the bottom of my heart.

Finally, this book would not have been possible without the unwavering support of my family. While I get the credit for shaping and changing laws and policies that make the world a better place, that's only possible because Ian has always given me the time, space and support to do what I want and what I feel needs to be done. Any achievements I have secured are also his. It simply would not have been possible without him. The same is true for my parents. Without their support, their care for our children when young, and then our dog when the children had left home, I would not have been able to carry on. Through reading about my work in the media and watching me on television, they've similarly had to live with insights into a world they would have preferred not to have. Yet they have always been resolute in their support.

I finally want to thank my children for bringing true joy to my life. They have both provided such valuable insights into the issues in this book, including reading and commenting on draft chapters. Talking to your mum about porn and sex is not easy, and probably not everyone's idea of parent–child conversations! What can I say, except thank you. This book is driven by my wish for my children, and any children they might have, to live in a better world. My generation has let your generation down. I know this book probably won't make much of a difference, but I write it in the hope that it just might. What else can I do?

Sources of Support

If you have been affected by any of the issues raised in this book, then please know you are not alone. Some key sources of support within the UK and worldwide are listed here. Most of these organisations also accept donations; visit their websites to find out more.

IN THE UK

Revenge Porn Helpline: Supports victim-survivors of image-based sexual abuse, including getting images and videos taken down from the internet – https://revengepornhelpline.org.uk/

StopNCII: A free tool that can help protect images being shared online by generating a digital fingerprint (not the image) that is then shared with social media and porn platforms – https://stopncii.org

Rape Crisis England and Wales: A feminist charity that offers counselling and support for those affected by rape and sexual violence – www.rapecrisis.org.uk

Rape Crisis Scotland: Supports those in Scotland affected by rape and sexual violence – https://www.rapecrisisscotland.org.uk/

Women's Aid: A charity dedicated to supporting women and girls, including those who are survivors of sexual violence – https://www.womensaid.org.uk/

Refuge: A specialist organisation that works with survivors of domestic abuse, as well as a specialist tech service for those affected by technology-facilitated abuse – https://refuge.org.uk/ and https://refugetechsafety.org/

#NotYourPorn: A movement that fights image-based sexual abuse. Website includes step-by-step guidance for victim-survivors of image-based sexual abuse – https://notyourporn.com

Safeline: A specialist sexual abuse support charity offering support and specialist helplines for women, men and non-binary and young people – https://safeline.org.uk/

SurvivorsUK: A specialist service for men, boys and non-binary people affected by sexual violence – https://www.survivorsuk.org/

Galop: A specialist organisation supporting LGBTQ+ victim-survivors of domestic and sexual abuse and hate crime – https://galop.org.uk/

End Violence Against Women Coalition: A coalition of 163 women's organisations from across the UK working to end violence against women and girls in all forms – https://www.endviolenceagainstwomen.org.uk/

SOURCES OF SUPPORT

NAPAC: Provides support for victim-survivors of childhood abuse – https://napac.org.uk/

Internet Watch Foundation: Works to prevent the repeated victimisation of those abused during childhood and removes child sexual abuse material online. You can report content – https://www.iwf.org.uk/

Lucy Faithfull Foundation: Supports anyone with a concern about child sexual abuse and its prevention, including men using child sexual abuse material or who have problematic porn use. Works with those concerned about others or their own behaviour – https://www.lucyfaithfull.org.uk/#about

Young Minds: Specialist mental health charity for young people – https://www.youngminds.org.uk/

Childline: Offers counselling and phoneline support for young people – https://www.childline.org.uk/get-support/

CEOP: Law enforcement agency working to protect children and young people from sexual exploitation and abuse, also takes reports of abuse – https://www.ceop.police.uk/safety-centre/

The Mix: A charity offering support and counselling for young people – https://www.themix.org.uk/get-support

Respond: A charity providing specialist support services to people with learning disabilities, autism or both who are victims of sexual abuse – https://respond.org.uk

Rights of Women: A charity providing support and legal advice to women experiencing all forms of violence and abuse – https://www.rightsofwomen.org.uk

National Stalking Helpline: Support and information for victims of stalking – https://www.suzylamplugh.org

WORLDWIDE

Revenge Porn Helpline Directory of Services: A directory of support available in many countries worldwide – https://revengepornhelpline.org.uk/how-can-we-help/if-we-can-t-help-who-can/help-for-victims-outside-the-uk/

Take It Down: Run by the Center for Missing and Exploited Children in the USA, and supports the anonymous removal of sexually explicit online content taken of children before they were eighteen – https://takeitdown.ncmec.org/

StopNCII.org: Operated by the Revenge Porn Helpline, this is a free tool that supports victim-survivors of intimate image abuse by creating digital fingerprints of images so they are easier to locate and remove – https://stopncii.org/

Cyber Civil Rights Initiative: Based in the USA, this organisation aims to combat online abuses that threaten civil rights and liberties. They operate both a bank of international resources and a directory of support – https://cybercivilrights.org/

SOURCES OF SUPPORT

In Hope: A global network of fifty-five organisations fighting against child sexual abuse online. In Hope also operates a directory detailing where to report image-based child sexual abuse in many different countries – https://www.inhope.org/EN

End Cyber Abuse: A global collective of lawyers and human rights activists working to end technology-facilitated gender-based violence. Fact sheets are available on their website explaining the law on image-based abuse in different countries – https://endcyberabuse.org/

Notes

INTRODUCTION

1. Han, C. et al. (2024), 'Characterizing the MrDeepFakes Sexual Deepfake Marketplace': https://arxiv.org/html/2410.11100v1.
2. Compton, S. and Hamlyn, R. (2023), 'The rise of deepfake pornography is devastating for women', CNN, 29 October 2023: https://edition.cnn.com/2023/10/29/opinions/deepfake-pornography-thriving-business-compton-hamlyn/index.html.
3. For discussions of patriarchy as it operates today, see Manne, K. (2017), *Downgirl: The Logic of Misogyny* (Oxford University Press) and Gilligan, K. and Snider, N. (2018), *Why Does Patriarchy Persist?* (Polity).
4. For an analysis of patriarchy and the role of men in pornography, see the pioneering work of Jensen, R. (2007), *Getting Off: Pornography and the End of Masculinity* (South End Press).
5. For a more in-depth discussion, see Eaton, A. (2007), 'A Sensible Antiporn Feminism', *Ethics*, 117, pp. 674–715.
6. While I focus on what I call patriarchal porn, others target what they characterise as 'inegalitarian pornography': see Eaton.
7. Rothman, E. (2021), *Pornography and Public Health* (Oxford University Press), p. vii.
8. See also Diana Russell, who contrasted pornography with erotica: Russell, D. (1994), *Against Pornography: the evidence of harm* (Russell Publications).
9. See further MacKinnon, C. (1987), *Feminism Unmodified* (Harvard University Press), p. 176.

10 Steinem, G. (1995; first published 1983), *Outrageous Acts and Everyday Rebellions* (Picador) p. 479.
11 There's a widely cited academic study that says that mainstream porn has not got 'harder and harder'. However, despite its popularity, this study is limited. It only spans 2008–16, and so cannot speak to recent changes in content. Also, the researchers were only able to examine around 250 videos, and even those were not representative. The researchers wanted to compare gay porn with heterosexual porn, as well as material involving performers from different ethnic backgrounds. These comparisons are valuable, and I discuss them in later chapters, but this does limit the sample. Indeed, the authors themselves say their findings must be taken cautiously when generalising about porn and aggression. See Shor, E. and Seida, K. (2018), '"Harder and Harder"? Is Mainstream Pornography Becoming Increasingly Violent and Do Viewers Prefer Violent Content?', *Journal of Sex Research*, 56(1), pp. 16–28.
12 Metha, M. and Plaza, D. (1997), 'Content Analysis of Pornographic Images Available on the Internet', *Information Society*, 13(2), pp. 153–61.
13 With notable exceptions, see Children's Commissioner (2023), *Evidence on pornography's influence on harmful sexual behaviour among children*, which talks about the 'violent themes' that were once on the 'margins' now being mainstream (p. 13): https://assets.childrenscommissioner.gov.uk/wpuploads/2023/05/Evidence-on-pornographys-influence-on-harmful-sexual-behaviour-among-children.pdf.
14 Gane, G., et al. (2024), 'Blurring the lines: the vague boundary between mainstream and deviant internet pornography tags for at-risk viewers', *Journal of Sexual Aggression*, 10(1), pp. 1–17.
15 Lucy Faithfull Foundation, 'When Porn Becomes a Problem', 6 March 2025: https://www.lucyfaithfull.org.uk/when-porn-becomes-a-problem/.

16 Ipsos Mori (2012), *A review of policy – sexual and sadistic violence in films – a report for the BBFC*: https://www.ipsos.com/sites/default/files/publication/0940-03/mediact_review%20sexual%20violence%20in%20movies.pdf.

17 Vera-Gray, F., et al. (2021), 'Sexual violence as a sexual script in mainstream online pornography', *British Journal of Criminology*, 61(5), pp. 1,243–60.

18 Gavey, N. (2018), *Just Sex? The Cultural Scaffolding of Rape* (2nd edn., Routledge).

19 Glitch UK (2023), *The Digital Misogynoir Report: ending the dehumanisation of Black women on social media*; and Glitch and ENAR, 'AI Deepfake Roundtable 1 Briefing', Glitch Research. Watch the roundtable here: https://glitchcharity.co.uk/our-work/ai-harms-redress.

20 Discussed in Burke, K. (2023), *The Pornography Wars: The Past, Present, and Future of America's Obscene Obsession* (Bloomsbury), p. 41.

21 Angel, K. (2021), *Tomorrow sex will be good again* (Verso), p. 27.

22 Gesselman, A., et al. (2024), 'The lifelong orgasm gap: exploring age's impact on orgasm rates', *Sexual Medicine*, 12(3). See also Piemonte, J., et al. (2019), 'Orgasm, gender, and responses to heterosexual casual sex', *Personality and Individual Differences*, 151 (109487).

23 Morgan, L. (2025), 'Bonnie Blue, Channel 4 and the problem with commodifying sexual violence', *Glamour*, 24 July 2025: https://www.glamourmagazine.co.uk/article/bonnie-blue-channel-4-1000-men-and-me.

24 Angel, K. (2021), *Tomorrow sex will be good again* (Verso), p. 28.

25 See Reeves, R. (2007), *John Stuart Mill: Victorian Firebrand* (Atlantic), p. 263, for a discussion of the harm principle and how *On Liberty* is often consciously 'misunderstood and misappropriated'. See also Richard Bellamy, who talks about how *On Liberty* is too frequently read in isolation and Mill's message is far more 'ambivalent' if we engage with the corpus of his work – Bellamy, R.

(1992), *Liberalism and Moral Society* (Pennsylvania State University Press), p. 22. This broader reading would include his works on women's subjection, as well as substantive analysis of issues such as domestic abuse and prostitution.

26 See further McGlynn, C. and Ward, I. (2014), 'Would John Stuart Mill have regulated pornography?', *Journal of Law and Society*, 41, pp. 500–22; Dyzenhaus, D. (1992), 'John Stuart Mill and the Harm of Pornography', *Ethics*, 102, p. 534.

27 For example, Mill advocated restrictions on those who had been convicted of offences while drunk in order to reduce the *risk* of future harms. See discussion in McGlynn and Ward, p. 507.

28 McGlynn, C. (2012), 'John Stuart Mill on Prostitution: Radical Sentiments, Liberal Proscriptions', *Nineteenth Century Gender Studies*, 8(2): https://www.ncgsjournal.com/issue82/mcglynn.html.

29 This draws on the ideas of liberal pragmatist Richard Rorty, who talked of the need for justice as a 'practical goal' rather than being based on 'abstract rights'. See McGlynn and Ward, (2009) 'Pornography, pragmatism and proscription', pp. *Journal of Law and Society,* 337–44.

30 Nussbaum, M. (2004), *Hiding from Humanity: digust, shame and the law* (Princeton University Press), pp. 139–47.

31 Legislative Scrutiny: (1) Criminal Justice and Courts Bill and (2) Deregulation Bill – Human Rights Joint Committee Contents, 11 June 2014: https://publications.parliament.uk/pa/jt201314/jtselect/jtrights/189/189.pdf.

32 Discussed in Craig, E. (2024), *Mainstreaming Porn* (McGill-Queen's University Press).

33 Brockhaus, H. (2022), 'Pope Francis: Pornography is "a threat to public health"', *Catholic News Agency*, 10 June 2022: https://www.catholicnewsagency.com/news/251512/pope-francis-pornography-is-a-threat-to-public-health.

34 Cole, S. (2025), 'Oklahoma Senator Introduces Bill to Make Porn Completely Illegal', *404 Media*, 27 January 2025: https://www.404media.co/oklahoma-senator-dusty-deevers-porn-bill/.

35 Norfolk, A. (2007), 'Jane Austen and the Case for Extreme Porn', *The Times*, 17 March 2007: https://www.thetimes.com/best-law-firms/profile-legal/article/jane-austen-and-the-case-for-extreme-porn-7wrtvcjh7bk?msockid=32ee36f6e23b64c7290720e6e38065bc.

36 Zahra Stardust, for example, does not claim that porn is *inherently* radical. See Stardust, Z. (2024), *Indie Porn: Revolution, Regulation, and Resistance* (Duke University Press).

I: BIG PORN

1 According to Pornhub, as reported by Cole, S. (2025), 'Pornhub Exec Discusses Pulling Out of the South, Trad Wives, and Feet Pics', *404 Media*, 27 January 2025: https://www.404media.co/podcast-pornhub-alexzandra-kekesi/.

2 Statistics and Data (2024), 'Most visited Websites – 1996/2023': https://statisticsanddata.org/data/most-visited-website-1996-2023/.

3 European Commission (2023), 'Commission designates second set of Very Large Online Platforms under the Digital Services Act', 20 December 2023: https://ec.europa.eu/commission/presscorner/api/files/document/print/en/ip_23_6763/IP_23_6763_EN.pdf.

4 Baker, L. (2020) 'Pornhub receives more website traffic than Amazon and Netflix, new research reveals!' *Business in the News*, 19 July 2020. Available at: https://businessinthenews.co.uk/2020/07/19/pornhub-receives-more-website-traffic-than-amazon-and-netflix-new-research-reveals/.

5 Ofcom (2023), 'Top trends from our latest look at people's online lives', 28 November 2023: https://www.ofcom.org.uk/media-use-and-attitudes/online-habits/top-trends-from-our-latest-look-at-peoples-online-lives/.

6 Statista (2023), 'Reach of online pornographic websites among male internet users in the UK in May 2023': https://www.statista.com/statistics/1473861/uk-reach-porn-websites-among-men/.

7 Statista (2024), 'DIGITAL & TRENDS: Online pornography in the UK': https://www.statista.com/study/171919/online-pornography-in-the-uk/.
8 Statista (2024), 'Worldwide visits to Pornhub from April 2022 to January 2024, by device': https://www.statista.com/statistics/1459714/pornhub-monthly-visits-by-device/.
9 Children's Commissioner (2023), '"A lot of it is actually just abuse": Young people and pornography': https://www.childrenscommissioner.gov.uk/resource/a-lot-of-it-is-actually-just-abuse-young-people-and-pornography/.
10 BBFC (2020), *Young people, Pornography & Age-verification*: https://www.revealingreality.co.uk/wp-content/uploads/2020/01/BBFC-Young-people-and-pornography-Final-report-2401.pdf.
11 5 Rights Foundation (2021), *Pathways: How digital design puts children at risk*: https://5rightsfoundation.com/wp-content/uploads/2021/09/Pathways-how-digital-design-puts-children-at-risk.pdf.
12 See Stardust, *Indie Porn: Revolution, Regulation, and Resistance.*
13 See Flory, I., et al. (2024), '"Porn is blunt [...] I had way more LGBTQ+ friendly education through porn": The experiences of LGBTQ+ individuals with online pornography', *Sexualities.*
14 There have been a series of investigations into some of the disturbing content on Only Fans, such as So, L., et al. (2024), 'Multiple OnlyFans accounts featured suspected child sex abuse, investigator reports', *Reuters*, 23 December 2024: https://www.reuters.com/investigates/special-report/onlyfans-sex-children-accounts/.
15 Kristof, N. (2020), 'The Children of Pornhub', *New York Times*, 4 December 2020: https://www.nytimes.com/2020/12/04/opinion/sunday/pornhub-rape-trafficking.html.
16 See Mickelwait, L. (2024), *Takedown: Inside the Fight to Shut Down Pornhub for Child Abuse, Rape, and Sex Trafficking* (Penguin Random House); and #NotYourPorn (2025): https://notyourporn.com/; and Mohan, M. (2020), 'I was raped at 14, and the video

ended up on a porn site', BBC News, 10 February 2020: https://www.bbc.co.uk/news/stories-51391981.
17. Kristof, N. (2024), 'Why Do We Let Corporations Profit from Rape Videos?', *New York Times*, 16 April 2024: https://www.nytimes.com/2021/04/16/opinion/sunday/companies-online-rape-videos.html.
18. Vera-Gray, F., et al., 'Sexual violence as a sexual script in mainstream online pornography'.
19. See Ethical Capital Partners (2023), 'ECP Announces Acquisition of MindGeek, Parent Company of Pornhub, 16 March 2023: https://www.ethicalcapitalpartners.com/news/ecp-announces-acquisition-of-mindgeek%2C-parent-company-of-pornhub; and Nilsson, P. (2023), 'Pornhub owner sold to Canadian private equity firm Ethical Capital', *Financial Times*, 16 March 2023: https://www.ft.com/content/69c3295e-6f45-4b5f-8e7b-3b8d56ca46c8.
20. As of July 2024, Pornhub was facing twenty-five lawsuits in relation to human trafficking, image-based sexual abuse, profiting from child sexual abuse material, and more. See Mickelwait, L. (2024), 'Pornhub Is Still a Crime Scene, Even After Its Rebrand', *Newsweek*, 23 July 2024: https://www.newsweek.com/pornhub-still-crime-scene-even-after-its-rebrand-opinion-1927282.
21. For example, Bonilla Muñiz, L. (2024), 'Attorney general, adult websites clash in age verification lawsuit', *News from the States*, 12 November 2024. Available at: https://www.newsfromthestates.com/article/attorney-general-adult-websites-clash-age-verification-lawsuit.
22. McCallum, S. and Vallance, C. (2024), 'Pornhub challenges EU over online content rules', BBC News, 7 March 2024: https://www.bbc.co.uk/news/technology-68500945.amp.
23. Horwitz, J. (2020), 'Facebook Executives Shut Down Efforts to Make the Site Less Divisive', *Wall Street Journal*, 26 May 2020: https://www.wsj.com/articles/facebook-knows-it-encourages-division-top-executives-nixed-solutions-11590507499.

24 Harris, T. (2016), 'How Technology is Hijacking Your Mind – from a Magician and Google Design Ethicist', *Medium*, 18 May 2016: https://medium.com/thrive-global/how-technology-hijacks-peoples-minds-from-a-magician-and-google-s-design-ethicist-56d62ef5edf3.

25 Zuboff, S. (2019), *The Age of Surveillance Capitalism: The Fight for a Human Future at the New Frontier of Power* (Profile Books).

26 Jaron Lanier, quoted in Zaman, M. (2020), 'The People Who Created Facebook & YouTube Are Sorry', *Refinery 29*, 2 September 2020: https://www.refinery29.com/en-us/2020/09/10002175/social-media-effects-the-social-dilemma-netflix-documentary.

27 Lanier, J. (2018), *Ten arguments for deleting your social media accounts* (Bodley Head).

28 Allen, M. (2017), 'Sean Parker unloads on Facebook: "God only knows what it's doing to our children's brains"', *Axios*, 9 November 2017: https://www.axios.com/2017/12/15/sean-parker-unloads-on-facebook-god-only-knows-what-its-doing-to-our-childrens-brains-1513306792.

29 Wells, G., et al. (2021), 'Facebook Knows Instagram Is Toxic for Teen Girls, Company Documents Show', *Wall Street Journal*, 14 September 2021: https://www.wsj.com/articles/facebook-knows-instagram-is-toxic-for-teen-girls-company-documents-show-11631620739.

30 Bryant, M. (2024), 'Instagram actively helping spread of self-harm among teenagers, study finds', *Guardian*, 30 November 2024: https://www.theguardian.com/technology/2024/nov/30/instagram-actively-helping-to-spread-of-self-harm-among-teenagers-study-suggests.

31 Zeynep Walton, A. (2025), *Logging Off: The Human Cost of Our Digital World* (Orion).

32 This section draws on: Adler, A. (2024), 'Arousal by Algorithm', *Cornell Law Review*, 109, pp. 787–842; Eaton, A. (2017), 'Feminist Pornography', in Mikkola M. (ed.) *Beyond Speech: Pornography*

and *Analytic Feminist Philosophy* (Oxford University Press), pp. 243–57; and Hanson, E. (2021), 'Pornography and Human Futures', *Fully Human*, p. 1.

33 As discussed in Vera-Gray, F. (2024), *Women on Porn: One hundred stories. One vital conversation* (Penguin), p. 15.

34 United States District Court, *Jane Doe vs MG Freesites Ltd*, 19 December 2024: https://endsexualexploitation.org/wp-content/uploads/Doe-1-et-al-v.-MG-Freesites-LTD-et-al_-MEMORANDUM-OF-OPINION-AND-ORDER-DENYING-CROSS-MOTIONS-FOR-SUMMARY-JUDGMENT-.pdf.

35 Mickelwait talks about ad impressions on her website, Trafficking Hub: https://lailamickelwait.com/traffickinghub/.

36 Craig, *Mainstreaming Porn*, p. 16.

37 Ibid, p. 18.

38 McDermott, S. (2025), 'Meta showed nearly 10,000 ads for deepfake clothes "erasing" app to Irish users since December', *The Journal*, 18 January 2025: https://www.thejournal.ie/ireland-nudify-app-ads-meta-deepfake-clothes-eraser-6594635-Jan2025/.

39 Garner, M. (2016), *Conflicts, contradictions and commitments: men speak about sexualisation of culture* (PhD, London Metropolitan University.)

40 Keilty, P. (2018), 'Desire by design: pornography as technology industry', *Porn Studies*, 5(3), pp. 338–42.

41 Stardust, p. 11.

42 Rama, I., et al. (2022), 'The platformization of gender and sexual identities: an algorithmic analysis of Pornhub', *Porn Studies*, 10(2), pp. 154–73.

43 For more on this, see Adler.

44 Aiston, J. (2021), 'What is the manosphere and why is it a concern?', Internet Matters, 4 October 2021: https://www.internetmatters.org/hub/news-blogs/what-is-the-manosphere-and-why-is-it-a-concern/.

45 Weiner, S. (2019), 'When YouTube Red-Pills the Love of Your Life', *Mel*, 19 January 2019: https://melmagazine.com/en-us/story/youtube-red-pill-men-right-wing-hate-radicalization.

46 Carpenter, S. (2024), 'Are "manfluencers" raising our sons?', CNN Health, 9 October 2024: https://edition.cnn.com/2024/10/09/health/manfluencers-raising-sons-wellness/index.html.

47 Das, S. (2022), 'Inside the violent, misogynistic world of TikTok's new star, Andrew Tate', *Guardian*, 6 August 2022: https://www.theguardian.com/technology/2022/aug/06/andrew-tate-violent-misogynistic-world-of-tiktok-new-star.

48 'The more you didn't like it, the more I enjoyed it. I fucking loved how much you hated it. It turned me on. ... Are you seriously so offended I strangled you a little bit? You didn't fucking pass out. Chill the fuck out, Jesus Christ.' Tate's words were released by *VICE World News* on X on 11 January 2023. The post had 2.8 million views and was used in a police investigation. See: https://x.com/VICEWorldNews/status/1613248602113179648.

49 Thomas, E. and Balint, K. (2022), 'Algorithms as a Weapon Against Women: How YouTube Lures Boys and Young Men into the "Manosphere"', Reset Australia: https://www.isdglobal.org/isd-publications/algorithms-as-a-weapon-against-women-how-youtube-lures-boys-and-young-men-into-the-manosphere/.

50 Ibid.

51 Baker, C., et al. (2024), *Recommending Toxicity: The role of algorithmic recommender functions on YouTube Shorts and TikTok in promoting male supremacist influencers*. DCU: https://fujomedia.eu/site/assets/files/2047/dcu-toxicity-full-report.pdf.

52 Spring, M. (2024), '"It stains your brain": How social media algorithms show violence to boys', BBC News, 2 September 2024: https://www.bbc.co.uk/news/articles/c4gdqzxypdzo.

53 See Campbell, R. (2024), 'Gender gap strongest at opposite ends of political spectrum in the 2024 General Election', King's College

London: https://www.kcl.ac.uk/news/gender-gap-strongest-at-opposite-ends-of-political-spectrum-in-the-2024-general-election.

54 Ipsos (2024), *Emerging tensions? How younger generations are dividing on masculinity and gender equality*, King's College London: https://www.kcl.ac.uk/policy-institute/assets/emerging-tensions.pdf.

55 Ibid.

56 Kahn, S. (2024), *Societal Threats and Declining Democratic Resilience: The New Extremism Landscape*, Crest Insights: https://www.crestadvisory.com/post/societal-threats-and-declining-democratic-resilience-the-new-extremism-landscape.

57 See Circle (2024), 'The Youth Vote in 2024: The Gender Gap: Young Women +17 for Harris, Young Men +14 for Trump': https://circle.tufts.edu/2024-election#youth-vote-+4-for-harris,-major-differences-by-race-and-gender.

58 Kurtzleben, D. (2024), 'How Trump and Vance's tour of dude influencers might help them win', NPR, 24 September 2024: https://www.npr.org/2024/09/20/g-s1-23911/how-trump-and-vances-tour-of-dude-influencers-might-help-them-win.

59 See Cokelaere, H. (2024), 'It's not just boomers, young people are voting far right too', *Politico*, 29 May 2024: https://www.politico.eu/article/europe-young-people-right-wing-voters-far-right-politics-eu-elections-parliament/.

60 Smith, S. (2024), 'How Reform UK won over so many Gen Z men', *Dazed*, 2 July 2024: https://www.dazeddigital.com/life-culture/article/63008/1/how-reform-uk-wooed-gen-z-men-britain-nigel-farage-general-election.

61 Read more in Bates, L. (2023), *Men who hate women: the extremism nobody is talking about* (Simon & Schuster).

62 Tranchese, A. and Sugiura, L. (2021), '"I Don't Hate All Women, Just Those Stuck-Up Bitches": How Incels and Mainstream Pornography Speak the Same Extreme Language of Misogyny', *Violence Against Women*, 27(14), pp. 2,709–34.

63 Johnson, A. (2010), 'To catch a curious clicker: A social network analysis of the online pornography industry', in Boyle, K. (ed.), *Everyday Pornography* (Routledge), pp. 159–75.
64 Gane, G., et al. (2024), 'Blurring the lines: the vague boundary between mainstream and deviant internet pornography tags for at-risk viewers', *Journal of Sexual Aggression*, 10(1), pp. 1–17.

2: HARMFUL PORN

1 BBC News Culture (2021), 'Billie Eilish says porn exposure while young caused nightmares', BBC News, 14 December 2021: https://www.bbc.co.uk/news/entertainment-arts-59658663#:~:text=Published,her percent20album percent 20Happier percent20Than percent20Ever.
2 Children's Commissioner (2023), '"A lot of it is actually just abuse": Young people and pornography': https://www.childrenscommissioner.gov.uk/resource/a-lot-of-it-is-actually-just-abuse-young-people-and-pornography/.
3 Ibid.
4 Gesselman, A., et al. (2024), 'The lifelong orgasm gap: exploring age's impact on orgasm rates', *Sexual Medicine*, 12(3). See also Piemonte, J., et al. (2019), 'Orgasm, gender, and responses to heterosexual casual sex', *Personality and Individual Differences*, 151 (109487).
5 Compton, J. (2019), 'The "orgasm gap": Why it exists and what women can do about it', NBC News, 6 April 2019: https://www.nbcnews.com/better/lifestyle/orgasm-gap-why-it-exists-what%02women-can-do-about-ncna983311.
6 Norris, S. (2024), '"Women believe that this is how they should be treated during sex" – is porn pressurising young women to expect sex that involves physical aggression?', *Stylist*: https://www.stylist.co.uk/relationships/porn-pressure-sexual-violence-aggression/943348.

7 Holden, M. (2021), 'These Gen Z Women Think Sex Positivity Is Overrated', Buzzfeed News, 21 July 2021: https://www.buzzfeednews.com/article/madeleineholden/gen-z-sex-positivity.
8 To read more about the development of the theory of 'sexual scripts' and its application to pornography, see my research with colleagues: Vera-Gray, F., et al., 'Sexual violence as a sexual script in mainstream online pornography'.
9 As discussed in Craig, *Mainstreaming Porn*, pp. 96–100.
10 See ibid, Chapter 4.
11 For a detailed discussion of this probability argument, see Eaton, 'A Sensible Anti-Porn Feminism', pp. 674–715.
12 For an early analogy between pollution and pornography, see Hynes, P. (1992), 'Pornography and Pollution: an environment analogy', in Itzin, C. (ed.), *Pornography: women, violence and civil liberties* (Oxford University Press), pp. 384–97.
13 My analysis borrows heavily from the thorough discussion in Eaton, pp. 674–715.
14 Casper, S., et al. (2025), 'Pitfalls of evidence-based AI Policy': https://arxiv.org/abs/2502.09618.
15 Eaton, A. (2017), 'Feminist pornography', in Mikkola, M. (ed.), *Beyond Speech: Pornography and Analytic Feminist Philosophy* (Oxford University Press), pp. 243–57.
16 Norris, S. (2024), '"Women believe that this is how they should be treated during sex" – is porn pressurising young women to expect sex that involves physical aggression?', *Stylist*: https://www.stylist.co.uk/relationships/porn-pressure-sexual-violence-aggression/943348.
17 BBFC (2020), *Young people, Pornography & Age-verification*: https://www.revealingreality.co.uk/wp-content/uploads/2020/01/BBFC-Young-people-and-pornography-Final-report-2401.pdf.
18 Children's Commissioner, '"A lot of it is actually just..."'.
19 Díaz-Moreno, A., Yupton Gómez, A., Bonilla, I., & Muro, A. (2025), 'Replication of Sexual Practices Depicted in Pornography

Among Spanish Youth: An Exploratory Study Based on Social Learning Theory', *Sexual Health & Compulsivity*, pp. 1–17.
20 Children's Commissioner (2023), *Evidence on pornography's influence on harmful sexual behaviour among children*: https://www.childrenscommissioner.gov.uk/resource/pornography-and-harmful-sexual-behaviour/.
21 Children's Commissioner, '"A lot of it is actually just abuse..."'.
22 See ibid and Children's Commissioner (2023), *Evidence on pornography's influence...*
23 Children's Commissioner, *Evidence on pornography's influence...*
24 Research with frontline workers suggests this is the case: The Behavioural Architects (2021), 'The relationship between pornography use and harmful sexual behaviours': https://www.gov.uk/government/publications/the-relationship-between-pornography-use-and-harmful-sexual-behaviours/the-relationship-between-pornography-use-and-harmful-sexual-attitudes-and-behaviours-literature-review; as did findings from an accompanying literature review.
25 Mori, C., et al. (2023), 'Exposure to sexual content and problematic sexual behaviors in children and adolescents: A systematic review and meta-analysis', *Child Abuse & Neglect*, 143: 106255.
26 Ybarra, M., et al. (2024), 'Predictors of the Onset of Sexual Violence Perpetration in Adolescence and Emerging Adulthood', *Prevention Science*, 25, pp. 1,284–97.
27 Children's Commissioner (2023), *Evidence on pornography's influence.*
28 See Ofsted (2021), *Review of sexual abuse in schools and colleges*, Gov.UK: https://www.gov.uk/government/publications/review-of-sexual-abuse-in-schools-and-colleges.
29 This is evident in the country reports prepared for the Council of Europe in its reviews of the implementation of the Istanbul Convention on Violence Against Women and Girls. See: https://www.coe.int/en/web/istanbul-convention/grevio.

30 van Oosten, J. and Vandenbosch, L. (2020), 'Predicting the Willingness to Engage in Non-Consensual Forwarding of Sexts: The Role of Pornography and Instrumental Notions of Sex', *Archives of Sexual Behaviour*, 49, pp. 1,121–32.
31 Marsh, W. (2024), '"The real thing almost didn't turn me on enough": how is online porn shaping the sex lives of young men?', *Guardian*, 27 January 2024: https://www.theguardian.com/society/2024/jan/28/australia-e-safety-commissioner-online-porn-study-data.
32 BBFC (2020), *Young people, Pornography & Age-verification*: https://revealingreality.co.uk/wp-content/uploads/2020/01/BBFC-Young-people-and-pornography-Final-report-2401.pdf.
33 Ofcom (2024), *Online Nation*: https://www.ofcom.org.uk/siteassets/resources/documents/research-and-data/online-research/online-nation/2024/online-nation-2024-report.pdf?v=386238.
34 Ibid.
35 Craig, E. (2024), *Mainstreaming Porn*, p. 33.
36 Vera-Gray, F. (2024), *Women on Porn: One hundred stories. One vital conversation* (Penguin).
37 See for example the work of Karen Boyle critiquing these debates back in 2000, Boyle, K. (2000), 'The Pornography debates: beyond cause and effect', *Women's Studies International Forum* 23, pp. 187–95.
38 Burnay, J., et al. (2022), 'Effects of violent and nonviolent sexualized media on aggression-related thoughts, feelings, attitudes, and behaviors: A meta-analytic review', *Aggressive Behavior*, 48, pp. 111–36.
39 Burnay, et al.
40 Herbenick, D., et al. (2020), 'Diverse Sexual Behaviors and Pornography Use: Findings from a Nationally Representative Probability Survey of Americans Aged 18 to 60 Years', *Journal of Sexual Medicine*, 17(4).
41 Krahé, B., et al. (2024), 'The role of pornography in shaping young adults' sexual scripts and sexual behavior: A longitudinal study with university students', *Psychology of Popular Media*.

42 The Behavioural Architects.
43 Ibid.
44 Wright, P. and Tokunaga, R. (2018), 'Women's perceptions of their male partners' pornography consumption and relational, sexual, self, and body satisfaction: toward a theoretical mode', *Annals of the International Communication Association*, 42(1), pp. 44–73.
45 See Rothman, *Pornography and Public Health*.
46 See ibid and Kelly, G. (2024), *Profits before people: How the pornography industry is normalising and monetising sexual violence*, CEASE: https://cease.org.uk/wp-content/uploads/2024/09/CEASE_Profits_Before_People_2024.pdf.
47 See Rothman.
48 See Rothman, and also Kelly.
49 McGlynn, C. and Rackley, E. (2009), 'Criminalising Extreme Pornography: A Lost Opportunity', *Criminal Law Review*, 4, pp. 245–60.
50 See this 2024 Italian study which confirms findings from other meta-analyses: Barchielli, B., et al. (2024), 'Exploring the Interplay of problematic pornography use, sexism, and rape myth acceptance: An Italian cross-sectional study', *Heliyon*, 10(13), e32981. See also Hedrick, A. (2021), 'A meta-analysis of media consumption and rape myth acceptance', *Journal of Health Communication*, 26(9), pp. 645–56.
51 Wang, S. and Kim, S. (2022), '"Users" emotional and behavioral responses to deepfake videos of K-pop idols', *Computers in Human Behavior*, 134, 107305.
52 Barchielli, et al.
53 Granada News (2022), 'Students campaign to stop school uniforms being sold in sex shops after being harassed in street', ITV News, 13 June 2022: https://www.itv.com/news/granada/2022-06-13/students-campaign-to-stop-school-uniforms-being-sold-in-sex-shops.

54 Children's Commissioner (2025), '"Sex is kind of broken now": children and pornography'.
55 Plan UK (2022), *'Everything is racialised on top': Black and minoritised girls' and young women's experiences of public sexual harassment in the UK*: https://plan-uk.org/sites/default/files/2023-05/Everything%20is%20Racialised%20Report.pdf.
56 Ibid, p. 19.
57 Jason Lanier makes the analogy between lead paint and social media in his 2018 book *Ten arguments for deleting your social media accounts*. I've adapted it for patriarchal porn.

3: ROUGH

1 Discussed in Herbenick, D., et al. (2021), 'What is rough sex, who does it and who likes it? Findings from a probability sample of US undergraduate students', *Archives of Sexual Behavior*, 50, pp. 1,183–95; Gavey, N. and Brewster, O. (2025), 'Is "Rough Sex" a Thing? A Survey of Meaning', *Journal of Sex Research*, pp. 1–17.
2 Herbenick, et al.
3 See Keane, S. (2023), 'Defining rough sex via mainstream pornography', in Bows, H. and Herring, J. (eds), *"Rough Sex" and the criminal law: global perspectives* (Emerald Publishing), pp. 53–68.
4 See Gavey, N. (2024) 'Deconstructing "Rough Sex" in a New Zealand Murder Trial: Beyond the Modern Mythology of Everyday Kink', *Social & Legal Studies*, pp. 1–22; Herbenick, et al.; Bows and Herring.
5 For brilliant analysis of this phenomenon, see Gavey, N. (2018), *Just Sex? The Cultural Scaffolding of Rape* (2nd edn, Routledge).
6 Gavey and Brewster.

7 Children's Commissioner (2023), '"A lot of it is actually just abuse"': https://www.childrenscommissioner.gov.uk/resource/a-lot-of-it-is-actually-just-abuse-young-people-and-pornography/.
8 Thompson, R. (2021), *Rough: how violence has found its way into the bedroom and what we can do about it* (Penguin).
9 See also Connellan, S. (2021), '*Mashable*'s Rachel Thompson investigates sexual violence (and what we can do about it) in *Rough*, Mashable, 26 August 2021: https://mashable.com/article/rachel-thompson-rough-sexual-violence-book.
10 Herbenick, D., et al. (2022), 'Frequency, Method, Intensity, and Health Sequelae of Sexual Choking Among U.S. Undergraduate and Graduate Students', *Archives of Sexual Behaviour*, 51, pp. 3,121–39.
11 See also Gavey, N. (2024), 'Deconstructing "Rough Sex" in a New Zealand Murder Trial: Beyond the Modern Mythology of Everyday Kink', *Social & Legal Studies*, pp. 1–22.
12 Mair, G. (2020), 'Over two-thirds of men under 40 have slapped, choked, gagged or spat on partner during sex', *Scottish Sun*, 23 March 2020: https://www.thescottishsun.co.uk/news/5415762/rough-sex-bbc-scotland-partner-men/.
13 Vogels, E. and O'Sullivan, L. (2019), 'The Relationship Among Online Sexually Explicit Material Exposure to, Desire for, and Participation in Rough Sex', *Archives of Sexual Behavior*, 48(2), pp. 653–65.
14 For a summary of all the recent studies, see Rothman, E. (2021), *Pornography and Public Health*, (Oxford University Press).
15 See Bridges, A., et al. (2010), 'Aggression and sexual behavior in best-selling pornography videos: A content analysis update', *Violence against Women*, 16(10), pp. 1,065–85; see also Rothman, p. 59.
16 See McKee, A. (2015), 'Methodological Issues in Defining Aggression for Content Analyses of Sexually Explicit Material', *Archives of Sexual Behavior*, 44(1), pp. 81–7; and the discussion of this study in Rothman, p. 59.

17 See further Rothman, p. 60, which draws on Shor, E. (2019), 'Age, Aggression, and Pleasure in Popular Online Pornographic Videos', *Violence Against Women*, 25(8), pp. 1,018–36.
18 See Fritz, N., et al. (2020), 'A descriptive analysis of the types, targets, and relative frequency of aggression in mainstream pornography', *Archives of Sexual Behavior*, 49(8), pp. 3,041–53. See also Carrotte, E., et al. (2020), 'Sexual Behaviors and Violence in Pornography: Systematic Review and Narrative Synthesis of Video Content Analyses', *Journal of Medical Internet Research*, 22(5): e16702.
19 Vera-Gray, et al. 'Sexual violence as a sexual script in mainstream online pornography'.
20 Lowbridge, C. (2020), 'Rough sex murder defence: Why campaigners want it banned', BBC News, 22 January 2020: https://www.bbc.co.uk/news/uk-england-51151182.
21 Engle, G. (2023), 'What is a spit kink? Here's everything you need to know', *Mashable*, 13 April 2023: https://mashable.com/article/spit-kink-sex-explained?test_uuid=01iI2GpryXngy77uIpA3Y4B&test_variant=a.
22 Discussed in Thompson, *Rough*, p. 75.
23 Thompson. See also Bows and Herring (2003), 'Rough sex', and Bows and Herring (2024), 'Non-Fatal Strangulation: An Empirical Review of the New Offence in England and Wales', *Journal of Criminal Law*, 88(5–6), pp. 332–46.
24 Gotell, L., et al. (2024), 'The Role of Pornography in the "Rough Sex" Defence in Canada', *Dalhousie Law Journal*, 47(2), p. 537.
25 See Faulkner, D. (2019), 'Grace Millane murder: A trial that gripped a nation', BBC News, 22 November 2019: https://www.bbc.co.uk/news/uk-england-essex-50515326; Gavey, N. (2024), 'Deconstructing "Rough Sex"…'.
26 Thompson, p. 80.
27 Quoted in ibid.
28 Perrone, P. (2008), 'Gerard Damiano: Director of the hugely successful porn film "Deep Throat"', *Independent*, 28 October 2008: https://

www.independent.co.uk/news/obituaries/gerard-damiano-director-of-the-hugely-successful-porn-film-deep-throat-976804.html.

29 See Thompson, p. 83.
30 Thompson, p. 83.
31 Shor, pp. 1,018–36.
32 Defer, A. (2022), 'Cum Tributes: Women Are Getting Harassed Online in a Gross New Way', *VICE*, 19 October 2022: https://www.vice.com/en/article/cum-tributes-gross-new-way-women-are-being-harassed-online/.
33 Thompson, R. (2020), 'How "hatewank" videos became a tool for harassing women in the public eye, *Mashable*, 7 July 2020: https://mashable.com/article/hatewank-videos-harassment?test_uuid=01iI2GpryXngy77uIpA3Y4B&test_variant=a.
34 Defer.
35 Ibid.
36 Thompson.
37 Lewis, R., et al. (2017), 'Heterosexual Practices Among Young People in Britain: Evidence from Three National Surveys of Sexual Attitudes and Lifestyles', *Journal of Adolescent Health*, 61(6), pp. 694–702; Herbenick, et al., 'Diverse Sexual Behaviors and Pornography Use: Findings from a Nationally Representative Probability Survey of Americans Aged 18 to 60 Years', pp. 623–33.
38 Gana, T. and Hunt, L. (2022), 'Young women and anal sex', *British Medical Journal*, p. 1,975: https://doi.org/10.1136/bmj.01975.
39 On the increasing prevalence of anal sex, see Herbenick, et al.
40 See for example, BBC News (2021), 'GirlsDoPorn victims win rights to their videos', BBC News, 17 December 2021: https://www.bbc.co.uk/news/technology-59699234; PA News Agency (2021), 'Pornhub sued by dozens of women alleging it profits from non-consensual content', *The National*, 18 June 2021: https://www.thenational.scot/news/national/19384497.pornhub-sued-dozens-women-alleging-profits-non-consensual-content/.

41 To read more of Anna's story, see McGlynn, C., et al. (2019), *Shattering Lives and Myths: A Report on Image-Based Sexual Abuse*: https://78cd5ee5-dd4a-48d2-ba03-9d4a490f335a.filesusr.com/ugd/e87dab_c6100ce67079407394dbb6100ebb937f.pdf.

42 I used Anna's phrasing as a title in an academic article, to convey the nature of the harms women experience. See McGlynn, C., et al. (2021), '"It's Torture for the Soul": The Harms of Image-Based Sexual Abuse', *Social & Legal Studies*, 30(4), pp. 541–62.

43 Moore, A. (2019), '"There's no end and no escape. You feel so, so exposed": life as a victim of revenge porn', *Guardian*, 22 September 2019: https://www.theguardian.com/lifeandstyle/2019/sep/22/theres-no-end-and-no-escape-you-feel-so-so-exposed-life-as-a-victim-of-revenge-porn. (Anna is referred to as Ruth in this article.)

44 Gane, G., et al. (2024), 'Blurring the lines: the vague boundary between mainstream and deviant internet pornography tags for at-risk viewers', *Journal of Sexual Aggression*, 10(1), pp. 1–17.

45 See NCOSE, *Not a Fantasy: how the pornography industry exploits image based sexual abuse in real life* (2025), p. 24.

46 Kingsley, T (2022), 'Online searches for "Ukrainian refugee porn" and "Ukrainian rape" surge 300 percent as Russian war rages', *Independent*, 27 May 2022: https://www.independent.co.uk/news/world/europe/ukraine-refugee-porn-rape-search-b2132402.html.

47 For a powerful discussion of this theme, see Garcia, M. (2023), *The Joy of Consent: A Philosophy of Good Sex* (Belknap Press).

48 Carrotte, E., et al. (2020), 'Sexual Behaviors and Violence in Pornography: Systematic Review and Narrative Synthesis of Video Content Analyses', *Journal of Medical Internet Research*, 22(5), e16702.

49 Discussed in Angel, p. 25.

4: COLOUR CODED

1 DiAngelo, R. (2016), *What does it mean to be white* (Counterpoints), p. 140.

2 Yin, L. and Sankin, A. (2020), 'Google Ad Portal Equated "Black Girls" with Porn', *The Markup*, 23 July 2020: https://themarkup.org/google-the-giant/2020/07/23/google-advertising-keywords-Black-girls.
3 Lorde, A. (2018), *The Master's Tools Will Never Dismantle the Master's House* (Penguin Classics).
4 See for example Imkaan, which describes itself as 'the UK's only national feminist umbrella organisation dedicated to addressing violence against Black and minoritised women and girls': https://www.imkaan.org.uk/. See also Milner, A., et al. (2020), 'Using the right words to address racial disparities in COVID-19', *Lancet Public Health*, 5(8), e419–e420.
5 Hirsch, A. (2018), '"As a black woman I'm always fetishised": racism in the bedroom', *Guardian*, 13 January 2018: https://www.theguardian.com/lifeandstyle/2018/jan/13/black-woman-always-fetishised-racism-in-bedroom.
6 Collins, P. H. (2000), *Black feminist thought: knowledge, consciousness and the politics of empowerment* (Routledge).
7 Walker, A. (1971), 'Coming apart', in *You Can't Keep a Good Woman Down* (Harcourt), p. 52.
8 Zheng, R. (2017), 'Race and pornography: the dilemma of the (un)desirable', in Mikkola, M. (ed.), *Beyond speech: pornography and analytic feminist philosophy* (Oxford University Press), pp. 177–96.
9 Lorde, A. (1984), *Sister Outsider* (Penguin Modern Classics), p. 54.
10 Gane, G., et al. (2024), 'Blurring the lines: the vague boundary between mainstream and deviant internet pornography tags for at-risk viewers', *Journal of Sexual Aggression*, 10(1), pp. 1–17.
11 Townsend, C. (2024), 'Why does the alt-right love interracial porn so much?', *Mashable*, 30 September 2024: https://mashable.com/article/right-wing-cuck-adult-content.
12 Samudzi, Z. (2018), 'What "Interracial" Cuckold Porn Reveals About White Male Insecurity', *VICE*, 31 July 2018: https://www.vice.com/en/article/interracial-cuckold-porn-white-male-insecurity-race/.
13 Ibid.

14 Townsend.
15 Shor, E. and Golriz, G. (2019), 'Race, and Aggression in Mainstream Pornography', *Archives of Sexual Behaviour*, 48, pp. 739–51.
16 Song, S. (2020), 'Meet the Couple Fighting Porn's Race Problem', *Paper*, 5 November 2020: https://www.papermag.com/royal-fetish-porn-race-problem#rebelltitem1.
17 Vera-Gray, *Women on Porn*, p. 103.
18 Shor and Golriz.
19 Fenton, S. (2015), 'The truth about pornography's race problem', *Independent*, 2 September 2015: https://www.independent.co.uk/news/world/americas/the-truth-about-pornography-s-race-problem-a6176986.html.
20 Vera-Gray, et al. 'Sexual violence as a sexual script in mainstream online pornography'.
21 Thompson, R. (2021), 'Porn, and porn sites, bolster racist tropes by design', *Mashable*, 10 September 2021: https://mashable.com/article/porn-racist-tropes.
22 On the jezebel stereotype and its links to slavery, see Pilgrim, D. (2024), 'The Jezebel Stereotype, Jim Crow Museum': https://jimcrowmuseum.ferris.edu/jezebel/index.htm.
23 On adultification, see Davis, J. (2022), 'Adultification bias within child protection and safeguarding', HM Inspectorate of Probation: https://hmiprobation.justiceinspectorates.gov.uk/document/adultification-bias-within-child-protection-and-safeguarding/.
24 See Cowan, G. and Campbell, R. (1994), 'Racism and Sexism in Interracial Pornography: A Content Analysis', *Psychology of Women Quarterly*, 18(3), pp. 323–38; Monk-Turner, E. and Purcell, H. (1999), 'Sexual violence in pornography: how prevalent is it?', *Gender Issues*, 17(2), pp. 58–67 and Fritz, N., et al. (2021), 'Worse Than Objects'.
25 Shor and Golriz.
26 Ibid.

27 Zhou, Y. and Paul, B. (2016), 'Lotus blossom or dragon lady: A content analysis of "Asian Women" online pornography', *Sexuality & Culture: An Interdisciplinary Quarterly*, 20(4), pp. 1,083–1,100.
28 Shor and Golriz.
29 Gossett, J. L., and Bryne, S. (2002), '"Click here": A content analysis of internet rape sites', *Gender & Society*, 16, pp. 689–709.
30 Nowrojee, S., and Silliman, J. (1997), 'Asian women's health: Organizing a movement', in Shah, S. (ed.), *Dragon ladies: Asian American feminists breathe fire*, (Sutherland Press), p. 78.
31 Mirzaei, Y., et al. (2022), 'Hijab Pornography: A Content Analysis of Internet Pornographic Videos', *Violence Against Women*, 28(6–7), pp. 1,420–40.
32 Ibid.
33 David Marchese, (2024), 'The Interview: Mia Khalifa's Messy World of Money, Sex And Activism', *New York Times*, 20 October 2024: https://www.nytimes.com/2024/10/19/magazine/mia-khalifa-interview.html.
34 de Oliveira, G., Slupska, J. (2023), *The Digital Misogynoir Report* (Glitch), p. 41.
35 Ibid., p. 42.
36 Zheng.
37 Vera-Gray, *Women on Porn*.
38 Discussed in Stardust, *Indie Porn*, p. 19.
39 See for example Miller-Young, M. (2014), *A taste for brown sugar: black women in pornography*, (Duke University Press); Nash, J. (2014), *The Black Body in Ecstasy: reading race, reading pornography*, (Duke University Press.)
40 Cited in Mayall, A., Russell, D. (1993), 'Racism in Pornography' in Diana Russell (ed) *Making Violence Sexy* (Open University Press) pp 167–177.
41 Vera-Gray, *Women on Porn*. pp. 98–9.

42 Ibid. p. 100.
43 Stardust, p. 11.
44 Samudzi.
45 Thompson.
46 Zheng.
47 Dickson, E. (2020), 'Racism in Porn Industry Under Scrutiny Amid Nationwide Protests', *Rolling Stone*, 10 June 2020: https://www.rollingstone.com/culture/culture-features/racism-porn-industry-protest-1010853/.
48 Thompson.
49 Cole, S. (2020), 'Fuck the Police: Why Does Cop Porn Still Exist?', *VICE*, 31 July 2020: https://www.vice.com/en/article/police-themed-cop-porn-rule-34/.
50 Ibid.
51 Thompson, pp. 160–1.
52 hooks, b. (1992), *Black Looks: Race and Representation* (Routledge p. 21.
53 Yin and Sankin.
54 See also the discussion in Keats Citron, D. (2022), *The Fight for Privacy: Protecting Dignity, Identity, and Love in the Digital Age* (Chatto & Windus), pp. 75–6.
55 Noble, S. (2018), *Algorithms of Oppression How Search Engines Reinforce Racism* (New York University Press).

5: BREATHLESS

1 Douglas, H., et al. (2024), 'Domestic Violence, Sex, Strangulation and the "Blurry" Question of Consent', *Journal of Criminal Law*, 88(1), pp. 48–66; and Bows and Herring, J. (2024), 'Non-Fatal Strangulation: An Empirical Review of the New Offence in England and Wales', pp. 332–46.
2 Rossen, R., et al. (1943), 'Acute arrest of cerebral circulation in man', *Archives of Neurology and Psychiatry*, 50(5).

3 Smith, B., et al. (2011), 'Experimental arrest of cerebral blood flow in human subjects: the red wing studies revisited', *Perspectives in Biology and Medicine*, 54(2).

4 The world-leading expert on the prevalence, impacts and societal challenges of sexual choking/strangulation is Debbie Herbenick, for details see: https://www.debbyherbenick.com/. Unless referenced otherwise, the data discussed in this chapter is from the multiple studies she's undertaken with colleagues. The key references are: Herbenick D., et al. (2023), 'Prevalence and characteristics of choking/strangulation during sex: Findings from a probability survey of undergraduate students', *Journal of American College Health*, 71(4), pp. 1,059–73; Herbenick, D., et al. (2022), '"It Was Scary, But Then It Was Kind of Exciting": Young Women's Experiences with Choking During Sex', *Archives of Sexual Behaviour*, 51, pp. 1,103–23; Herbenick, D., et al. (2020), 'Diverse Sexual Behaviors and Pornography Use: Findings from a Nationally Representative Probability Survey of Americans Aged 18 to 60 Years', *Journal of Sexual Medicine*, 17(4), pp. 623–33; Herbenick, D., et al. (2022), 'Frequency, Method, Intensity, and Health Sequelae of Sexual Choking Among U.S. Undergraduate and Graduate Students', *Archives of Sexual Behaviour*, 51, pp. 3,121–39; Herbenick, D., et al. (2022), 'Non-Fatal Strangulation/Choking During Sex and Its Associations with Mental Health: Findings from an Undergraduate Probability Survey', *Journal of Sex and Marital Therapy*, 48(3), pp. 238–50; Herbenick, D., et al. (2023), '#ChokeMeDaddy: A Content Analysis of Memes Related to Choking/Strangulation During Sex', *Archives of Sexual Behavior*, 52, pp. 1,299–1,315.

5 Sharman, L. S., et al. (2024), 'Strangulation During Sex Among Undergraduate Students in Australia: Toward Understanding Participation, Harms, and Education', *Sexuality Research and Social Policy*.

6 Schori, A., et al. (2022), 'How Safe Is BDSM?: A Literature Review on Fatal Outcome in BDSM Play', *International Journal of Legal*

Medicine, 136(1), pp. 287–95; Hone, J. (2024), '"I think it's natural": why has sexual choking become so prevalent among young people?', *Guardian*, 1 September 2024: https://www.theguardian.com/lifeandstyle/article/2024/sep/02/i-think-its-natural-why-has-sexual-choking-become-so-prevalent-among-young-people.

7 Discussed in Herbenick, et al., '"It Was Scary, But Then It Was Kind of Exciting"', and Sharman, et al., 'Strangulation during sex among undergraduate students'.

8 Laan, E. T. M., Klein, V., Werner, M. A., van Lunsen, R. H. W., Janssen E. (2021), 'In Pursuit of Pleasure: A Biopsychosocial Perspective on Sexual Pleasure and Gender', *International Journal of Sexual Health*, 33(4), pp. 516–36.

9 See Hou, J., et al. (2023), 'Structural brain morphology in young adult women who have been choked/strangled during sex: A whole-brain surface morphometry study', *Brain Behaviour*, 13(8), e3160; Huibregtse, M., et al. (2022), 'Frequent and Recent Non-fatal Strangulation/Choking During Sex and Its Association With fMRI Activation During Working Memory Tasks', *Frontiers in Behavioral Neuroscience*, 16, 881678.

10 Sharman, et al., 'Strangulation during sex among undergraduate students'.

11 Palys, T. (1986), 'Testing the common wisdom: The social content of video pornography', *Canadian Psychology*, 27(1), pp. 22–5.

12 Bridges, A., et al. (2010), 'Aggression and sexual behavior in best-selling pornography videos: A content analysis update', *Violence against Women*, 16(10), pp. 1,065–85.

13 See Fritz, N. (2020), 'A descriptive analysis of the types, targets, and relative frequency of aggression in mainstream pornography', *Archives of Sexual Behavior*, 49(8), pp. 3,041–53, which was a study of content on porn sites from 2013 to 2014.

14 Erika Lust, one of the few women porn producers, discusses the normalisation of violence in mainstream porn in Moore, A., Khan, C. (2019), 'The fatal, hateful rise of choking during sex', *Guardian*,

25 July 2019: https://www.theguardian.com/society/2019/jul/25/fatal-hateful-rise-of-choking-during-sex.
15 Péloquin, T. (2023), 'Pornography – a kind of rape education', Lapresse, 10 June 2023: https://www.lapresse.ca/actualites/2023-06-10/pornographie/une-sorte-d-education-au-viol.php.
16 Wright, P, et al. (2023), 'Pornography Consumption and Sexual Choking: An Evaluation of Theoretical Mechanisms', *Health Communication*, 38(6), pp. 1,099–1,110.
17 Sharman, L., et al. (2024), 'Prevalence of sexual strangulation/choking among Australian 18–35 year olds', *Archives of Sexual Beahvior*.
18 Bonnar, M. (2020), 'I thought he was going to tear chunks out of my skin', BBC News Scotland, 23 March 2020: https://www.bbc.co.uk/news/uk-scotland-51967295.
19 Wright, et al.
20 Vogels, E. and O'Sullivan (2019), 'The Relationship Among Online Sexually Explicit Material Exposure to, Desire for, and Participation in Rough Sex', *Archives of Sexual Behavior*, 48(2), pp. 653–65.
21 Sharman, et al.
22 Smailes, H. and McGowan, M. (2024), *Strangulation During Consensual Sex in the UK: A report on findings from a pilot survey conducted in October 2024*, Institute for Addressing Strangulation, Bangor University: https://ifas.org.uk/wp-content/uploads/2024/12/Strangulation-During-Sex-in-the-UK-December-2024-FINAL.pdf.
23 Harte, A. (2019), 'A man tried to choke me during sex without warning', BBC News, 28 November 2019: https://www.bbc.co.uk/news/uk-50546184.
24 Herbenick; Vilhjálmsdóttir, A., Forberg, T. (2023), *Sexual asphyxia: The state of choking during sex in Iceland* (Doctoral dissertation, Reykjavik University): https://skemman.is/bitstream/1946/44608/1/The%20state%20of%20choking%20during%20sex%20in%20Iceland.pdf.

25 See Mair, G. (2020) 'Seven in ten men have had "rough sex"', *The Times*, 23 March 2020: https://www.thetimes.com/uk/scotland/article/seven-in-ten-men-have-had-rough-sex-jh9hvc98j?msockid=32ee36f6e23b64c7290720e6e38065bc; Bonnar, 'I thought he was going to tear chunks out of my skin'.
26 Smailes and McGowan, *Strangulation During Consensual Sex in the UK*.
27 For a powerful discussion of sexual choking/strangulation, see Thompson, *Rough*, p. 61.
28 Sharman, et al; Herbenick, et al., '"It Was Scary, But Then It Was Kind of Exciting".
29 Marocico, O. and Milne, B. (2024), '"Tate raped and strangled us" – women talk to BBC', BBC News, 9 September 2024: https://www.bbc.co.uk/news/articles/cwyje823er4o.
30 Sentencing Council (2025), 'Strangulation or suffocation / Racially or religiously aggravated strangulation or suffocation', Sentencing Council: https://sentencingcouncil.org.uk/guidelines/strangulation-or-suffocation-racially-or-religiously-aggravated-strangulation-or-suffocation/.
31 Sharman, L., et al. (2024), 'Prevalence of Sexual Strangulation/Choking'; Sharman, L., et al. (2024), 'Strangulation during sex'.
32 Norris, S. (2024), '"Women believe that this is how they should be treated during sex" – is porn pressurising young women to expect sex that involves physical aggression?', *Stylist*: https://www.stylist.co.uk/relationships/porn-pressure-sexual-violence-aggression/943348.
33 See further Angel, *Tomorrow sex will be good again*.
34 Quoted in Romito, P. (2008), *A deafening silence: Hidden violence against women and children* (Policy Press), p. 151.

6: BARELY LEGAL

1 Das, S. (2019), 'Unilever and Heinz pay for ads on Pornhub, the world's biggest porn site', *The Sunday Times*, 3 November 2019:

https://www.thetimes.com/article/unilever-and-heinz-pay-for-ads-on-pornhub-the-worlds-biggest-porn-site-knjzlmwzv.
2. See Mohan, M. (2020), 'I was raped at 14, and the video ended up on a porn site'; Lati, M. (2021), 'Pornhub profits from rape, child pornography and sex trafficking, dozens of women allege in lawsuit', *Washington Post*, 18 June 2021: https://www.washingtonpost.com/business/2021/06/18/pornhub-lawsuit-rape-child-porn-sex-trafficking/.
3. See Lapsia, S. (2024), *Tech Platforms Used by Online Child Sexual Abuse Offenders: Research Report with Actionable Recommendations for the Tech Industry*, Protect Children: https://www.suojellaanlapsia.fi/en/post/tech-platforms-child-sexual-abuse.
4. Lapsia.
5. Cited in ibid, p. 7.
6. National Crime Agency News (2020), 'European police chiefs back NCA demands for tech companies to do more to prevent child sex abuse, National Crime Agency, 14 February 2020: https://www.nationalcrimeagency.gov.uk/news/european-police-chiefs-back-nca-demands-for-tech-companies-to-do-more-to-prevent-child-sex-abuse.
7. In 2023, the Stanford Internet Observatory published a report where they found 'large-scale communities' sharing paedophilia content on Instagram. See Levine, A. (2022), 'These TikTok Accounts Are Hiding Child Sexual Abuse Material in Plain Sight', *Forbes*, 14 November 2022: https://www.forbes.com/sites/alexandralevine/2022/11/11/tiktok-private-csam-child-sexual-abuse-material/. See also Camber, R. (2024), 'Instagram "is profiting from AI-generated child abuse images"', *Daily Mail*, 22 July 2024: https://www.dailymail.co.uk/news/article-13657395/Instagram-faces-legal-challenge-claims-social-media-giant-profits-allowing-users-advertise-AI-generated-child-sex-abuse-images.html.

8   So, L., et al. (2024), 'Multiple OnlyFans accounts featured suspected child sex abuse, investigator reports', *Reuters*, 23 December 2024: https://www.reuters.com/investigates/special-report/onlyfans-sex-children-accounts/.
9   Vera-Gray, et al., 'Sexual violence as a sexual script in mainstream online pornography'.
10 Gane, et al., 'Blurring the lines: the vague boundary between mainstream and deviant internet pornography tags for at-risk viewers', pp. 1–17.
11 Shor, E. (2019), 'Age, Aggression, and Pleasure in Popular Online Pornographic Videos', *Violence Against Women*, 25(8), pp. 1,018–36.
12 Shor.
13 See Dines, G. (2011), *Pornland: How Porn Has Hijacked Our Sexuality* (Beacon Press).
14 See Gail Thackray's blog post on starting *Barely Legal* magazine: Thackray, G. (2019), 'Starting *Barely Legal* Magazine, Running with wolves': https://www.runningwithwolvesbook.com/post/starting-barely-legal-magazine.
15 Morrish, L. (2024), 'Ads for Explicit "AI Girlfriends" Are Swarming Facebook and Instagram', *Wired*, 25 April 2024: https://www.wired.com/story/ads-for-explicit-ai-girlfriends-swarming-facebook-and-instagram/.
16 Gane, G., et al. (2024). See also 'Instagram "Most Important Platform" for Child Sex Abuse Networks: Report', *Globe Post*, 28 June 2023: https://theglobepost.com/2023/06/09/instagram-child-sex-abuse-platform/; and Tiel, D and Diresta, R. (2023), 'Child safety on federated social media', Stanford Internet Observatory, Cyber Policy Centre, 24 July 2023: https://purl.stanford.edu/vb515nd6874.
17 Grant, H., '"I didn't start out wanting to see kids in porn": are porn algorithms feeding a generation of paedophiles – or creating one?', *Guardian*, 5 April 2025: https://www.theguardian.com/society/2025/

apr/05/i-didnt-start-out-wanting-to-see-kids-are-porn-algorithms-feeding-a-generation-of-paedophiles-or-creating-one.

18 Prichard, J., et al. (2022), 'Online messages to reduce users' engagement with child sexual abuse material: A review of relevant literature for the reThink chatbot', UCL Discovery: https://discovery.ucl.ac.uk/id/eprint/10152516/.

19 Gane, et al.

20 Brown, S. (2023), 'Key messages from research on child sexual abuse by adults in online contexts', Centre of Expertise on Child Sexual Abuse: https://www.csacentre.org.uk/app/uploads/2023/10/Key-messages-from-research-on-child-sexual-abuse-by-adults-in-online-contexts-ENGLISH.pdf. See also Hamilton, M. and Belton, I. (2022), 'Offences Involving Indecent Images of Children: Literature Review', Scottish Sentencing Council: https://www.scottishsentencingcouncil.org.uk/media/1jbb3w4l/indecent-images-of-children-literature-review.pdf; and Rimer, J. and Holt, K. (2023) '"It was in control of me": Notions of addiction and online child sexual exploitation material offending', *Sexual Abuse*, 35(1), pp. 3–30.

21 See Gane, G., et al. (2024), and Knack, N., et al. (2020), 'Motivational pathways underlying the onset and maintenance of viewing child pornography on the Internet', *Behavioural Sciences and the Law*, 38(2), pp. 100–16.

22 Lapsia.

23 Jay, A., et al. (2022), *The Report of the Independent Inquiry into Child Sexual Abuse*, p. 212: https://www.iicsa.org.uk/key-documents/31216/view/report-independent-inquiry-into-child-sexual-abuse-october-2022_0.pdf.

24 Insoll, T., et al. (2022), 'Risk Factors for Child Sexual Abuse Material Users Contacting Children Online: Results of an Anonymous Multilingual Survey on the Dark Web', *Journal of Online Trust and Safety*, 1(2), pp. 1–24.

25 Salter, M., et al. (2023), *Identifying and understanding child sexual offending behaviours and attitudes among Australian men*, p. 31: https://www.humanrights.unsw.edu.au/news/worlds-largest-child-sexual-abuse-perpetration-prevalence-study-recommends-significant-investment-early-intervention-measures.
26 Ibid.
27 Cubitt, T., et al. (2024), 'The overlap between viewing child sexual abuse material and fringe or radical content online', Australian Institute of Criminology: https://doi.org/10.52922/ti77710.
28 Children's Commissioner, '"A lot of it is actually just abuse"...'.
29 For a global perspective, see Unicef (2024), 'Over 370 million girls and women globally subjected to rape or sexual assault as children': https://www.unicef.org/press-releases/over-370-million-girls-and-women-globally-subjected-rape-or-sexual-assault-children. For England and Wales specifically, see Office for National Statistics (2023), *Sexual offences victim characteristics, England and Wales: year ending March 2022*: https://www.ons.gov.uk/peoplepopulationandcommunity/crimeandjustice/articles/sexualoffencesvictimcharacteristicsenglandandwales/yearendingmarch2022.
30 See further the national reports of the monitoring body of the Council of Europe Istanbul Convention on Violence Against Women and Girls, available at https://www.coe.int/en/web/istanbul-convention/latest-evaluation-reports-and-evaluation-visits. See for example Austria's report: GREVIO (2024), *Building trust by delivering support, protection and justice Austria First thematic evaluation report*, p. 9: https://rm.coe.int/first-thematic-evaluation-report-building-trust-by-delivering-support-/1680b18c17.
31 See United States District Court (2024), *Jane Doe vs MG Freesites Ltd*, p. 10: https://endsexualexploitation.org/wp-content/uploads/Doe-1-et-al-v.-MG-Freesites-LTD-et-al_-MEMORANDUM-OF-

OPINION-AND-ORDER-DENYING-CROSS-MOTIONS-FOR-SUMMARY-JUDGMENT-.pdf.

32 Ibid., p. 9.
33 Ibid.
34 Kristof.
35 Read more in Mickelwait, *Takedown: Inside the Fight to Shut Down Pornhub for Child Abuse, Rape, and Sex Trafficking.*
36 Kristof, N. (2025), 'These internal documents show why we shouldn't trust porn companies', *New York Times*, 10 May 2025: https://www.nytimes.com/2025/05/10/opinion/pornhub-children-documents.html?unlocked_article_code=1.Gk8.XYOt.FIbocJLyhTB_&smid=url-share.
37 Lucy Faithfull Foundation (2024), 'Pioneering chatbot reduces searches for illegal sexual images of children': https://www.lucyfaithfull.org.uk/pioneering-chatbot-reduces-searches-for-illegal-sexual-images-of-children/.
38 Scanlan J, Prichard J, Hall LC, Watters P, Wortley R, (2024) 'reThink Chatbot Evaluation', (University of Tasmania, Hobart).
39 Ibid.
40 Prichard, et al. (2022).
41 Prichard, et al. (2022).
42 Leake, N. (2024), 'Ofcom apologises over "ill-judged" pornography LinkedIn post', *Telegraph*, 17 December 2024: https://www.telegraph.co.uk/news/2024/12/17/ofcom-apologises-linkedin-job-advert-pornography/.

7: FAMILY TIES

1 This chapter is indebted to the research of Janine Benedet and Isabel Grant on child sexual abuse and incest, particularly, Benedet, J. and Grant, I. (2020), 'Breaking the Silence on Father–Daughter Sexual Abuse of Adolescent Girls: A Case Law Study', *Canadian Journal of Women and the Law*, 32(2), pp. 239–87.

2 Discussed in Herman, J. and Hirschman, L. (1981), *Father–Daughter Incest* (Harvard University Press), p. 737.
3 Bender, L. and Blau, A. (1937), 'The reaction of children to sexual relations with adults', *American Journal of Orthopsychiatry*, 7(4), pp. 500–18.
4 Cormier, B., et al. (1962), 'Psychodynamics of Father Daughter Incest', *The Canadian Journal of Psychiatry*, 7(5), pp. 203–17.
5 Herman and Hirschman.
6 As discussed in Benedet and Grant.
7 Stroebel, S., et al. (2012), 'Father–Daughter Incest: Data from an Anonymous Computerized Survey', *Journal of Child Sexual Abuse*, 21(2), pp. 176–99, see pp. 177–8.
8 Beard, K., et al. (2017), 'Father-Daughter Incest: Effects, Risk-Factors, and a Proposal for a New Parent-Based Approach to Prevention', *Sexual Addiction and Compulsivity*, 24(1–2), pp. 79–107.
9 Azman, U., et al. (2024), 'Breaking the silence: underlying factors influencing father-daughter incest survivors', *International Journal of Studies on Children, Women, Elderly and Disabled*, 20, pp. 97–104.
10 Azman, et al.
11 Child Safeguarding Practice Review Panel (2024), '"I wanted them all to notice": Protecting children and responding to child sexual abuse within the family environment', UK Government, p. 21: https://assets.publishing.service.gov.uk/media/67446a8a81f809b32c8568d3/CSPRP_-_I_wanted_them_all_to_notice.pdf.
12 HM Government (2021), *Tackling Child Sexual Abuse Strategy*: https://assets.publishing.service.gov.uk/government/uploads/system/uploads/attachment_data/file/973236/Tackling_Child_Sexual_Abuse_Strategy_2021.pdf.
13 Ibid, p. 27.
14 Benedet and Grant.
15 98 percent of perpetrators are men in the most recent study of child sexual abuse: Child Safeguarding Practice Review Panel (2024).
16 Benedet and Grant.

17 See discussion of the Pornhub video *giving step-daddy her virginity for step-father's day* in Craig, *Mainstreaming Porn*, pp. 118–19.
18 The harrowing nature of these experiences which are so often dismissed, is discussed in Kelly, L. (1988), *Surviving Sexual Violence* (Polity).
19 Strong, F. (2022), 'Acknowledge, address, adapt', RCEW: https://www.sarsas.org.uk/wp-content/uploads/2022/03/SARSAS-SSAP-Policy-Report_10037_1.6.pdf.
20 Relva, I., et al. (2017), 'Dyadic Types of Sibling Sexual Coercion', *Journal of Family Violence*, 32, pp. 577–83.
21 Strong.
22 Yates, P. and Allardyce, S. (2021), *Sibling sexual abuse: A knowledge and practice overview*, Centre of Expertise on Child Sexual Abuse: https://www.csacentre.org.uk/app/uploads/2023/09/Sibling-sexual-abuse-report.pdf.
23 For a trenchant critique of our current malaise on child sexual abuse, read: 'Ignore the stigma and tackle the toxic cycle of child sexual abuse', *Guardian*, 30 November 2024: https://www.theguardian.com/commentisfree/2024/nov/30/the-observer-view-ignore-the-stigma-and-tackle-the-toxic-cycle-of-child-sexual-abuse.
24 Child Safeguarding Practice Review Panel and *Observer* (30 November 2024).
25 My focus is also on porn produced for the male heterosexual market. There is, however, much incestuous porn in sections of the mainstream sites labelled as 'gay porn'. See discussion in Craig, *Mainstreaming Porn*, pp. 119–20.
26 Herman, p. 25.
27 Ibid.
28 Palys, T. (1986), 'Testing the common wisdom: The social content of video pornography', *Canadian Psychology*, 27(1), pp. 22–5.
29 Metha Dwaine Plaza, M. (1997), 'Content Analysis of Pornographic Images Available on the Internet', *The Information Society*, 13(2), pp. 153–61.

30 Rothman, *Pornography and Public Health*, p.54.
31 Ibid and O'Neil, L. (2018), 'Incest Is the Fastest Growing Trend in Porn. Wait, What?', *Esquire*, 28 February 2018: https://www.esquire.com/lifestyle/sex/a18194469/incest-porn-trend/.
32 Morczek, A. (2018), 'Eroticizing Intrafamilial Sexual Violence', *Family & Intimate Partner Violence Quarterly*, 10(3), pp. 65–71.
33 See O'Neil, L. (2018), 'Incest Is the Fastest Growing Trend in Porn. Wait, What?', and Brown, V. (2016), 'Breaking taboos: Incest pornography is becoming more popular and *Game of Thrones* could be to blame', *The Sun*, 11 June 2016: https://www.thesun.co.uk/living/1268468/incest-pornography-is-becoming-more-popular-and-game-of-thrones-could-be-to-blame/. For a thorough critique of the arguments using *Game of Thrones* as a reason why not to take incest porn seriously, see Craig, particularly Chapter 5.
34 O'Neil, L. (2018), 'Incest Is the Fastest Growing Trend in Porn. Wait, What?'.
35 Talbot, H. (2019), *Breaking Down Porn: A Classification Office Analysis of Commonly Viewed Pornography in NZ*, NZ Office of Film and Literature Classification: https://www.classificationoffice.govt.nz/media/documents/Breaking_Down_Porn.pdf.
36 See Craig, Chapter 5.
37 Similar titles include 'Don't Tell My Mother' and 'redhead teen is messing with her stepfather into fucking her'.
38 Naftulin, J. and Mendez II, M. (2021), '"Incest" influencers are crushing it on social media, using taboo tropes to amass followers. It's a classic porn-industry move', *Business Insider*, 3 May 2021: https://uk.style.yahoo.com/incest-influencers-crushing-social-media-150000352.html.
39 Lefebvre, A. (2025), 'Why is incest porn so insanely popular right now?', *The Daily Beast*, 29 January 2025: https://www.thedailybeast.com/why-is-step-incest-porn-so-insanely-popular-right-now/.

40 See also discussion in Craig.
41 Pornhub (2023), *2023 Transparency Report (First Half)*, Pornhub Help Center: https://help.pornhub.com/hc/en-us/articles/46213033364371-2023-Transparency-Report-First-Half.
42 Lefebvre.
43 Craig, p22.
44 Talbot, p. 7.
45 Martijn, F., et al. (2020), 'A meta-analysis comparing male adolescents who have sexually offended against intrafamilial versus extrafamilial victims', *Clinical Child and Family Psychology Review*, 23(4), pp. 529–52.
46 Michael Slater et al. (2023), *Identifying and understanding child sexual offending behaviours and attitudes among Australian men*: https://www.humanrights.unsw.edu.au/news/worlds-largest-child-sexual-abuse-perpetration-prevalence-study-recommends-significant-investment-early-intervention-measures.
47 Craig.
48 Ibid, p. 127.
49 Romito, *A deafening silence: Hidden violence against women and children*.

8: WITHOUT CONSENT

1 Serrato, J. (2022), 'SD fugitive on FBI's 'Most Wanted List' captured in Spain', Fox 5 News, 23 December 2022: https://fox5sandiego.com/news/local-news/sd-fugitive-on-fbis-most-wanted-list-captured-in-spain/.
2 Cole, S. (2019), 'Girls Do Porn Goes to Trial Over Allegations Women Were Tricked into Videos', *VICE*, 28 June 2019: https://www.vice.com/en/article/girls-do-porn-goes-to-trial-over-allegations-women-were-tricked-into-videos/.

3 Gault, M. and Cole, S. (2021), 'Girls Do Porn' Victims Reach Settlement with Pornhub, VICE, 16 October 2021: https://www.vice.com/en/article/girls-do-porn-victims-reach-settlement-with-pornhub/.
4 Eastern District of New York (2023), 'Pornhub Parent Company Admits to Receiving Proceeds of Sex Trafficking and Agrees to Three-Year Monitoring', 21 December 2023: https://www.justice.gov/usao-edny/pr/pornhub-parent-company-admits-receiving-proceeds-sex-trafficking-and-agrees-three-year.
5 US Attorney's Office: Southern District of California (2024), 'GirlsDoPorn Owner Michael Pratt Extradited to Face Sex Trafficking Charges', 19 March 2024: https://www.justice.gov/usao-sdca/pr/girlsdoporn-owner-michael-pratt-extradited-face-sex-trafficking-charges.
6 Cole, S. (2023), 'Girls Do Porn Victims Say Cloudflare Participates in 'Criminal Venture' by Servicing Sites That Host Videos of Their Abuse', VICE, 27 April 2023: https://www.vice.com/en/article/girls-do-porn-victims-cloudflare/.
7 Burges, M. (2024), 'Deepfake Creators Are Revictimizing GirlsDoPorn Sex Trafficking Survivors', Wired, 25 June 2024: https://www.wired.com/story/girlsdoporn-deepfake-victim-videos/.
8 Cole, S., et al. (2020), '"Frankenstein's Monster": Images of Sexual Abuse Are Fueling Algorithmic Porn', VICE, 10 November 2020: https://www.vice.com/en/article/sexual-abuse-fueling-ai-porn-deepfake-czech-casting-girls-do-porn/.
9 See Thiel, D. (2023), 'Identifying and Eliminating CSAM in Generative ML Training Data and Models', Stanford Digital Repository: https://purl.stanford.edu/kh752sm9123.
10 Bose, A. (2024), 'Kathua to Kolkata: The Internet Is Obsessed with Rape Videos, Decode', Decode, 26 August 2024: https://

www.boomlive.in/decode/kolkata-doctor-rape-murder-why-is-the-internet-obsessed-with-rape-porn-videos-26291.

11 Noor, A. (2024), Kolkata Rape & Murder: Searches for Victim's 'Video' Trend on Google, Porn Sites, *The Quint*, 20 August 2024: https://www.thequint.com/gender/kolkata-rape-murder-rg-kar-hospital-searches-for-victims-video-trend-on-google-porn-sites.

12 Ross, T. (2013), Online porn: animals have more rights than women, campaigners say, *The Telegraph*, 18 June 2013: https://www.telegraph.co.uk/news/politics/10126161/Online-porn-animals-have-more-rights-than-women-campaigners-say.html.

13 McGlynn, C. and Bows, H. (2019), 'Possessing Extreme Pornography: Policing, Prosecutions and the Need for Reform', *The Journal of Criminal Law*, 83(6), pp. 473–88.

14 Herbenick, et al. (2020), 'Diverse Sexual Behaviors and Pornography Use: Findings from a Nationally Representative Probability Survey of Americans Aged 18 to 60 Years', *Journal of Sexual Medicine*, 17(4): 623–33.

15 Children's Commissioner (2025), '"Sex is kind of broken now": children and pornography'.

16 Roberts, Y. (2025), '"DIY swab kits? It's better than doing nothing": the controversial scheme to tackle rape on campus', *Guardian*, 16 February 2025: https://www.theguardian.com/society/2025/feb/16/diy-swab-kits-scheme-campus-rape.

17 Davis, K. (2019), '"Stealthing": Factors Associated with Young Men's Nonconsensual Condom Removal', *Health Psychology*, 38(11), pp. 997–1,000.

18 Moore, A. (2021), 'The sexual assault of sleeping women: the hidden, horrifying rape crisis in our bedrooms', *Guardian*, 15 June 2021: https://www.theguardian.com/society/2021/jun/15/the-sexual-assault-of-sleeping-women-the-hidden-horrifying-crisis-in-britains-bedrooms.

19 Moore, A. (2024), 'The horror and history of drug-facilitated rape: "When I woke up my body felt battered"', *Guardian*, 20 November 2024: https://www.theguardian.com/society/2024/nov/20/the-truth-about-drug-facilitated-rape.
20 Dodd, V. (2025), 'UCL student accused tells court he liked pornography featuring sleeping women', *Guardian*, 25 February 2025: https://www.theguardian.com/uk-news/2025/feb/17/ucl-student-accused-of-tells-court-he-liked-pornography-featuring-sleeping-women.

9: DEEPFAKED

1 Cole, S. (2017), 'AI-Assisted Fake Porn Is Here and We're All Fucked', *VICE*, 11 December 2017: https://www.vice.com/en/article/gal-gadot-fake-ai-porn/.
2 Harwell, D. (2018), 'Scarlett Johansson on fake ai generated sex videos: 'Nothing can stop someone cutting and pasting my image', *Washington Post*, 31 December 2018: https://www.washingtonpost.com/technology/2018/12/31/scarlett-johansson-fake-ai-generated-sex-videos-nothing-can-stop-someone-cutting-pasting-my-image/.
3 Guy, J. (2023), 'Outcry in Spain as artificial intelligence used to create fake naked images of underage girls', CNN, 20 September, 2023: https://edition.cnn.com/2023/09/20/europe/spain-deepfake-images-investigation-scli-intl/index.html.
4 Thompson, D. (2023), 'Girl pupils "at risk" after an alarming rise in "toxic masculinity" in schools, *Scottish Mail on Sunday*, 3 December 2023: https://www.dailymail.co.uk/news/article-12818177/Girl-pupils-risk-alarming-rise-toxic-masculinity-schools.html.
5 Chandran, R. (2023), 'Flood of AI and deepfake images underline threat to women, sexual minorities in South Asia', Scroll.in, 16 December 2023: https://scroll.in/article/1060585/flood-of-ai-and-

deepfake-images-underline-threat-to-women-sexual-minorities-in-south-asia.

6   BBC News (2022), 'Two arrested in Egypt after teenage girl's suicide sparks outrage', BBC News, 4 January 2022: https://www.bbc.co.uk/news/world-middle-east-59868721. Hooper, S. (2024), 'Girl killed herself when bullies shared fake nudes of her', *Metro*, 24 January 2024: https://metro.co.uk/2024/01/24/teen-took-life-online-bullying-shared-fake-nudes-20162284/.

7   Ajder, H., et al. (2019), 'The State of Deepfakes: Landscape, Threats, and Impact', Deeptrace: https://regmedia.co.uk/2019/10/08/deepfake_report.pdf.

8   Cole, 'AI-Assisted Fake Porn Is Here and We're All Fucked'.

9   Read more in Cole, S. (2023), *How Sex Changed the Internet and the Internet Changed Sex* (Workman Publishing Company).

10 Iozzio, C. (2016), 'The Playboy Centrefold That Helped Create the JPEG', *The Atlantic*, 9 February 2016: https://www.theatlantic.com/technology/archive/2016/02/lena-image-processing-playboy/461970/.

11 As set out in the San Fransico legal case: https://www.courthousenews.com/wp-content/uploads/2024/08/nudify-websites-lawsuit.pdf.

12 MyImageMyChoice, *Deepfake abuse – landscape analysis* (2023): https://myimagemychoice.org/take-action/#issue.

13 Burgess, M. (2024), 'Millions of People Are Using Abusive AI "Nudify" Bots on Telegram', *Wired*, 15 October 2024: https://www.wired.com/story/ai-deepfake-nudify-bots-telegram/.

14 West, K. (2024), 'I was deepfaked by my best friend', BBC News, 2 April 2024: https://www.bbc.co.uk/news/uk-68673390.

15 Davies, J. (2025), *No-one wants to see your dick: a handbook for survival in the digital world* (Headline Publishing).

16 Glitch (2023), 'Roundtables on AI harms: Deepfake Abuse & Non-Criminal Redress': https://glitchcharity.co.uk/our-work/ai-harms-redress.

17 Hodgson, C. (2015), 'Controversial porn star Mia Khalifa is receiving death threats for wearing a hijab', *Cosmopolitan*, 7 January 2015: https://www.cosmopolitan.com/uk/entertainment/news/a32392/porn-star-mia-khalifa-death-threats/

18 Mort, H. (2023), 'I felt numb – not sure what to do. How did deepfake images of me end up on a porn site?', *Guardian*: https://www.theguardian.com/technology/2023/oct/28/how-did-deepfake-images-of-me-end-up-on-a-porn-site-nfbntw.

19 Sohal, B. (2023), 'Do British Asian Women think Deepfakes will increase Revenge Porn?', Deziblitz, 15 December 2023: https://www.desiblitz.com/content/do-british-asian-women-think-deepfakes-will-increase-revenge-porn.

20 Chesney, R. and Citron, D. (2018), 'Deep Fakes: A Looming Challenge for Privacy, Democracy, and National Security', *California Law Review*, 107, pp. 1,753–1,820.

21 Morgan, L. (2024), 'Cally Jane Beech: "Image-based abuse is a pandemic against women and girls"', 1 October 2024: https://www.glamourmagazine.co.uk/article/cally-jane-beech-interview-2024-glamour-women-of-the-year-awards.

22 Dickson, E. (2020), 'TikTok Stars Are Being Turned Into Deepfake Porn Without Their Consent', *Rolling Stone*, 26 October 2020: https://www.rollingstone.com/culture/culture-features/tiktok-creators-deepfake-pornography-discord-pornhub-1078859/.

23 Morris, A. (2022), 'Cara Hunter MLA: Stress of fake clip made my life absolutely horrific in election run-up', *Belfast Telegraph*, 9 May 2022: https://www.belfasttelegraph.co.uk/news/northern-ireland/cara-hunter-mla-stress-of-fake-clip-made-my-life-absolutely-horrific-in-election-run-up/41629366.html.

24 Ayyub, R. (2018), 'I Was the Victim of a Deepfake Porn Plot Intended to Silence Me', *Huffington Post*, 21 November 2018: https://www.huffingtonpost.co.uk/entry/deepfake-porn_uk_5bf2c126e4b0f32bd58ba316.

25 For more on Kate's and Cara's stories, watch the NZZ documentary *Fake Porn, Real Victims*: Krättli, N. (2021), *Fake Porn – Real*

Victims. How women become targets of AI, NZZ, 1 September 2021: https://www.nzz.ch/english/video-fake-porn-real-victims-how-women-become-targets-of-artificial-intelligence-ld.1754001. I'm also in the documentary commenting on the unacceptable lack of legal action to tackle these abuses.

26 Oppenheim, M. (2022), 'I discovered deepfake porn of myself online', Independent, 25 November 2022: https://www.independent.co.uk/news/uk/home-news/deepfakes-porn-downblousing-crime-b2232913.html.

27 The documentary is available to watch here: BBC Three (2023), *Deepfake Porn: Could You Be Next?*, BBC, 5 January 2023: https://www.bbc.co.uk/programmes/m001c1mt. See also Hastings, C. (2022), 'BBC Three's Deepfake Porn: Could You Be Next? explores the terrifying rise of image-based sexual abuse', *Stylist*, January 2022: https://www.stylist.co.uk/entertainment/deepfake-porn-you-could-be-next-bbc-three-release-date/704652.

28 Edinburgh University (2023), 'Addressing the Issue: revenge porn and deepfakes', Girl Up podcast, 22 November 2023: https://open.spotify.com/episode/4Foz4WuAij3JfUA95e5ho5.

29 McGlynn, C. (2024), 'Deepfake porn: why we need to make it a crime to create it, not just share it', *The Conversation*, 9 April 2024: https://theconversation.com/deepfake-porn-why-we-need-to-make-it-a-crime-to-create-it-not-just-share-it-227177.

30 Vera-Gray, F. (2018), *The right amount of panic: how women trade freedom for safety* (Policy Press).

31 Read more in McGlynn, C. and Tuna Toparlak, (2025), 'The New Voyeurism: criminalising the creation of "deepfake porn"', *Journal of Law and Society*. 52(2): 204-228.

32 Cox, J. (2024), 'Someone Put Facial Recognition Tech onto Meta's Smart Glasses to Instantly Dox Strangers', 404, 2 October 2024: https://www.404media.co/someone-put-facial-recognition-tech-onto-metas-smart-glasses-to-instantly-dox-strangers/.

33 Cole, 'AI-Assisted Fake Porn ...'.

10: VIRTUAL REALITIES

1. Discussed in Craig, *Mainstreaming Porn*, pp.14–15.
2. Bedbible Research Centre (2024), VR Porn Industry Statistics, 14 May 2024: https://bedbible.com/vr-porn-industry-statistics/.
3. Institute of Engineering and Technology (2022), Safeguarding the Metaverse: https://www.theiet.org/media/9836/safeguarding-the-metaverse.pdf.
4. Dupré, M. (March 2024), 'Meta's VR Headsets Are Getting a Masturbation Mode', *Futurism*, 13 March 2024: https://futurism.com/the-byte/metas-vr-headsets-masturbation-mode.
5. See for example William, R. (2024), 'How to Watch VR Porn on Apple Vision Pro (Tutorial)', ARVR Tips, 4 September 2024: https://arvrtips.com/how-to-watch-vr-porn-on-apple-vision-pro/.
6. Roblox (2024), 'Roblox Reports Third Quarter 2024 Financial Results', 31 October 2024: https://ir.roblox.com/news/news-details/2024/Roblox-Reports-Third-Quarter-2024-Financial-Results/default.aspx.
7. See Hinduja, S., Patchin, J. (2024) 'Metaverse Risks and Harms among US Youth: Experiences, Gender Differences, and Prevention and Response Measures', New Media & Society.
8. Institute of Engineering and Technology (2022).
9. See Bedbible (2024), VR Porn Industry Statistics, 14 May 2024: https://bedbible.com/vr-porn-industry-statistics/.
10. Stanney, K. et al (2020), 'Virtual Reality Is Sexist: But It Does Not Have to Be', *Frontiers*, 31 January 2020, 7(4), doi: 10.3389/frobt.2020.00004.
11. See Sample, I. (2022) '"Virtual reality is genuine reality" so embrace it, says philosopher', *Guardian*, 17 January 2022: https://www.theguardian.com/technology/2022/jan/17/virtual-reality-is-genuine-reality-so-embrace-it-says-us-philosopher.
12. See McCallum, S. (2022), 'Tool to spot breast cancer at home wins UK Dyson award', BBC News, 7 September 2022: https://www.bbc.co.uk/news/technology-62807367.

13 Bates, L. (2025), *The New Age of Sexism* (Simon Schuster), p. 148.
14 Pornhub (2018) Year in Review: https://www.pornhub.com/insights/2018-year-in-review.
15 Elsey, J., et al. (2019), 'The impact of virtual reality versus 2D pornography on sexual arousal and presence', *Computers in Human Behaviour*, 1(97), pp. 35–43.
16 Dekker, A., et al. (2020), 'VR Porn as "Empathy Machine"? Perception of Self and Others in Virtual Reality pornography', *The Journal of Sex Research*, 58(3), pp. 273–8.
17 Simon, S. and Greitemeyer, T. (2019), 'The impact of immersion on the perception of pornography: A virtual reality study', *Computers in Human Behaviour*, 93, pp. 141–8.
18 Dekker, et al.
19 Brown, N., et al. (2023), 'Exploring Women's State-Level Anxiety in Response to Virtual Reality Erotica', *Journal of Sex & Marital Therapy*, 50(2), pp. 137–51.
20 Milk, C. (2015), 'How virtual reality can create the ultimate empathy machine', TED, 1 March 2015: https://www.ted.com/talks/chris_milk_how_virtual_reality_can_create_the_ultimate_empathy_machine.
21 Read more about this in Myers, M. (no date), 'The empathy machine? Virtual reality and the search for a solution to violence', *Griffith Review*: https://www.griffithreview.com/articles/the-empathy-machine/.
22 Helmore, E. (2015), '"Godmother of VR" sees journalism as the future of virtual reality', *Guardian*, 11 March 2015: https://www.theguardian.com/technology/2015/mar/11/godmother-vr-news-reporting-virtual-reality. See also Myers; and Nonny de la Peña's TED talk on virtual reality and the news: De la Peña, N. (2015), 'The future of news? Virtual reality', TED, May 2015: https://www.ted.com/talks/nonny_de_la_pena_the_future_of_news_virtual_reality.
23 See Watson, Z. (2017), 'VR for News: The New Reality?', Reuters Institute: https://reutersinstitute.politics.ox.ac.uk/sites/default/files/research/files/VR%2520for%2520news%2520-

%2520the%2520new%2520reality.pdf. and Messeri, L. (2024), *In the Land of the Unreal: Virtual and Other Realities in Los Angeles* (Duke University Press).

24 Cummings (2024), 'Assessing virtual reality's value as an "empathy machine"', Yale News, 15 May 2024: https://news.yale.edu/2024/05/15/assessing-virtual-realitys-value-empathy-machine. See also the University of Barcelona's research into the use of VR with domestic violence perpetrators (2016), 'Virtual reality improves offenders' empathy', *Science Daily*, 16 February 2016: https://www.sciencedaily.com/releases/2018/02/180226090915.htm. Also Seinfeld, S., et al. (2021), 'Being the victim of virtual abuse changes default mode network responses to emotional expressions', *Cortex*, 135, pp. 268–84.

25 Sora-Domenjó, C. (2022) 'Disrupting the "empathy machine": The power and perils of virtual reality in addressing social issues', *Frontiers in Psychology*, 26(13).

26 Dekker, et al.

27 This statement can be found on the front page of the sex emulator website.

28 Riess makes the point that empathy is not always an 'equal opportunity benefactor'. See Riess, H. (2017), 'The Science of Empathy', *Journal of Patient Experience*, 4(2), pp. 74–7.

29 Younger men with higher incomes and sexual minorities report more frequent engagement with all forms of sextech: Gesselman, A., et al. (2022), 'Engagement with emerging forms of sextech: demographic correlates from a national sample of adults in the United States', *Journal of Sex Research*, 3, pp. 1–3.

30 See further Sora-Domenjó, C. (2022) 'Disrupting the "empathy machine": The power and perils of virtual reality in addressing social issues', *Frontiers in Psychology*, 26(13).

31 Myers.

32 Martingano, A. (2021), 'Virtual reality improves emotional but not cognitive empathy: A meta-analysis', *Technology, Mind, and Behaviour*, 2(6).

33 Sherry Turkle quoted in Mineo, L. (2023), 'Why virtual isn't actual, especially when it comes to friends', *Harvard Gazette*, 5 December 2023: https://news.harvard.edu/gazette/story/2023/12/why-virtual-isnt-actual-especially-when-it-comes-to-friends/.
34 See Reeves, C. (2011), 'Fantasy depictions of child sexual abuse: The problem of age play in Second Life', *Journal of Sexual Aggression*, 19(2), pp. 236–46 and Reeves, C. (2018), 'The virtual simulation of child sexual abuse: online gameworld users' views, understanding and responses to sexual age play', *Ethics and Information Technology*, 20(2), pp. 101–13.
35 Pettifer, S., et al. (2022), 'The Future of eXtended Reality Technologies, and Implications for Online Child Sexual Exploitation and Abuse', University of Manchester: https://documents.manchester.ac.uk/DocuInfo.aspx?DocID=62042 and https://documents.manchester.ac.uk/display.aspx?DocID=62042.
36 UWE Bristol (2023), 'New research reveals how virtual reality poses significant risk to children', 5 September 2023: https://www.uwe.ac.uk/news/new-research-reveals-virtual-reality-poses-significant-risk-to-children.
37 Pettifer, et al.
38 Cole, S. and Maiberg, E. (2019), '"They Can't Stop Us": People Are Having Sex With 3D Avatars of Their Exes and Celebrities', *VICE*, 19 November 2019: https://www.vice.com/en/article/they-cant-stop-us-people-are-having-sex-with-3d-avatars-of-their-exes-and-celebrities/.
39 Cole and Maiberg.
40 Discussed in Pettifer, et al.
41 For a very prescient discussion of the effects of emerging tech including virtual reality, see Franks, M. (2009), 'Unwilling Avatars: Idealism and Discrimination in Cyberspace', *Columbia Journal of Gender and Law*, 20, p. 224.
42 As anticipated in this study: Wood, M., et al. (2017), '"They're Just Tixel Pits, Man": Disputing the "Reality" of Virtual Reality pornography through the Story Completion Method', in 2017 CHI Conference on

Human Factors in Computing Systems, Human Factors in Computing Systems, Denver, Colorado, USA, pp. 5,439–51.
43 Pettifer, et al.
44 See Arrell and colleague's discussion of the potential benefits of sex tech and new technologies, though concerns are also noted: Arrell, R., et al. (2022), 'Sex and Emergent Technologies', in *Routledge Handbook of Philosophy of Sex and Sexuality* (Routledge), pp. 586–600.

11: HOW WE FIGHT BACK

1 Kleeman, J. (2018), 'YouTube star wins damages in landmark UK "revenge porn" case', *Guardian*, 17 January 2018: https://www.theguardian.com/technology/2018/jan/17/youtube-star-chrissy-chambers-wins-damages-in-landmark-uk-revenge-porn-case.
2 Chrissy's story, including us speaking at the 2015 event, are captured in this video by Jenny Kleeman for the *Guardian* (3 June 2015): https://www.theguardian.com/uk-news/video/2015/jun/03/revenge-porn-chrissy-chambers-justice-video
3 *FGX v Gaunt* (27 February 2023): https://www.judiciary.uk/wp-content/uploads/2023/02/FGX-v-Gaunt-Judgment-270223.pdf. See also Castro, B. (28.02.2023), 'First "revenge porn" civil case sees judge award £100,000', *Law Society Gazette*: https://www.lawgazette.co.uk/news/first-revenge-porn-civil-case-sees-judge-award-100000/5115274.article.
4 Walker, P. (2023), 'Georgia Harrison's £200k damages over Stephen Bear sex tape', BBC News, Essex, 26 July 2023: https://www.bbc.co.uk/news/uk-england-essex-66319446.
5 For a compelling and disturbing account of the myriad ways technology, including chatbots, are being used to abuse and harass women, see Bates, *The New Age of Sexism*.
6 See further McGlynn, C. (2024), 'Towards a New Criminal Offence of Intimate Intrusions', *Feminist Legal Studies*, 32, pp. 189–212.

7   Wegerstad, L. (2021), 'Theorising sexual harassment and criminalisation in the context of Sweden', *Bergen Journal of Criminal Law and Criminal Justice*, 9(2), pp. 61–81.
8   See McGlynn, C. (2025), 'Why incest porn is more common and harmful than you think' *The Conversation*, 27 February 2025: https://theconversation.com/why-incest-porn-is-more-common-and-harmful-than-you-think-247512.
9   Woods, L. (2024), 'Ofcom's approach to human rights in the illegal harms consultation', Online Safety Act Network, 1 February 2024: https://www.onlinesafetyact.net/analysis/ofcoms-approach-to-human-rights-in-the-illegal-harms-consultation/.
10 ASA and CAP (2024), 'ASA Ruling on Metamind AI Ltd t/a AI Persona', ASA CAP, 11 December 2024: https://www.asa.org.uk/rulings/metamind-ai-ltd-a24-1251099-metamind-ai-ltd.html.
11 French Senate report (2022), *Porn: Hell behind the scenes*: https://www.senat.fr/rap/r21-900-1/r21-900-1.html. See also Cease (2025), *Profits before People: how the porn industry is normalising and monetising sexual violence*.
12 Independent Review of Pornography (Bertin Review) (2025), Creating a safer world: the challenge of regulating online pornography: https://www.gov.uk/government/publications/creating-a-safer-world-the-challenge-of-regulating-online-pornography and https://assets.publishing.service.gov.uk/media/67c0802016dc9038974dbc71/HC_592_The_Challenge_of_Regulating_Online_Pornography.pdf.
13 Rothman, *Pornography and Public Health*, especially chapters 11 and 12 on trafficking and the conditions of the industry.
14 Ibid.
15 Discussed in McGlynn, A. (2021), 'Feminist Pornography as Feminist Propaganda, and Ideological Catch-22s', in J. Lackey (ed.), *Applied Epistemology* (Oxford Academic), pp. 283–301.
16 Read more in Taormino, T., et al. (eds) (2013), *The Feminist Porn Book, The Politics of Producing Pleasure* (The Feminist Press Cuny).

17 Stardust, *Indie Porn*. See also Berg, H. (2021), *Porn Work – sex, labor and late capitalism* (University of North Carolina Press).
18 Ryberg, I. (2015), 'Imagining a safe space in feminist pornography', in L. Mulvey and A. Blackman Rogers (eds), *Feminisms: diversity, difference and multiplicity in contemporary film cultures* (Amsterdam University Press), pp. 79–85.
19 McGlynn, 'Feminist Pornography as Feminist Propaganda'.
20 See Eaton, 'Feminist Pornography', pp. 243–57.
21 McGlynn.
22 Vera-Gray, *Women on Porn*.
23 Rose, K. and Mustafa, T. (2025), '10 ethical porn sites that are inclusive and empowering', *Glamour*, 3 February 2025: https://www.glamourmagazine.co.uk/article/best-ethical-porn-sites#intcid=_glamour-uk-right-rail_69fb8670-b924-4c17-b25f-43f571eb3166_popular4-1.
24 See Cindy Gallop's Ted Talk, 'Make love, not porn' (February 2009): https://www.ted.com/talks/cindy_gallop_make_love_not_porn; and her interview with Sophie Browner: Browner, S. (2016), 'There Are No Royalties in Porn: An Interview with Cindy Gallop, CEO of Make Love Not Porn', *Los Angeles Review of Books*, 16 November 2016: https://lareviewofbooks.org/article/no-royalties-porn-interview-cindy-gallop-ceo-make-love-not-porn/.
25 See further End Violence Against Women and Girls, 'New RHSE Guidance' https://www.endviolenceagainstwomen.org.uk/new-rshe-guidance-to-address-porn-misogyny-and-vawg/.
26 See further: https://www.beyondequality.org/.

CONCLUSION: RECLAIMING
SEXUAL FREEDOM AND DESIRE

1 Discussed in Angel, *Tomorrow sex will be good again*, p. 67.
2 Craig, *Mainstreaming Porn*, p. 22.

NOTES

3   This argument was first most clearly put forward by Catharine MacKinnon (1993), *Only Words* (Harvard University Press).
4   Read more in Srinivasan, A. (2020), *The Right to Sex* (Bloomsbury).
5   Franks, M. (2024), *Fearless Speech: breaking free of the first amendment* (Bold Type Books).
6   Beard M. (2017), *Women and Power: a manifesto* (Profile Books), quoted in Franks, p. 36.

Index

3D 12, 197, 200–14
'4-foot-6 porn' 124–5, 136
4chan 185

Abigail (on being choked) 117
'actual bodily harm' 108
Advertising Standards Authority, UK 234
advertising, targeted 32, 35, 55, 199, 200, 212
'affection-based' incest 145–6, 159
age-assurance laws 58, 229–30
aggression 73–5, 96, 97–8, 132, 138
AI (artificial intelligence):
   AI-manipulated masculinity 38–9
   child sexual abuse 226
   generative 12, 14, 185
   girlfriends 129
   Google and 103
   incest 234
   inter-governmental summit 227
   sexualised deepfakes 2–3, 11–12, 164, 180–99
   See also virtual-reality porn
Al Adib, Miriam 181–2
algorithms 32, 33, 36–8, 93–5, 100, 132, 135, 154, 196
'ambiguous' consent 62, 122–3

anal sex 81–2, 173
animalistic depiction 93, 95, 97
anime, explicit 94
Anna ('image-based sexual abuse') 84–5
Apple 201
arousal 244–6
BDSM 76
child porn 133
choking/strangulation 110
family ties 11, 48–50
non-consent 177
normal 232
porn and 86–7, 99
virtual-reality 200, 204–6, 208, 209, 211, 213–14
Asian people 65
Asian women/girls 91, 97–8, 100, 127, 190
'asphyxiation' 105–23
assault, physical 96, 108
assault, sexual:
   consent and 79
   intrafamilial 138, 157
   survivor experiences 188–9
   teens and 59–60, 133
   university campuses 172
   while asleep 49, 51

INDEX

See also individual offences
augmented reality 197, 212
Australia 30, 33–4, 114, 115–16, 162, 225
avatars 197, 200–1, 203–4, 209–13, 221–2
Aylo (porn company) 26, 31
Ayyub, Rana 192, 196

Barbie (2023 film) 122
Barely Legal magazine 128–9
'barely legal' porn 28, 65, 74, 124–40
Barraclough, Louise 82–3
Bates, Laura 204
BBC:
   investigations 40, 116, 117, 139, 186
   Deepfake Porn: Could You Be Next? 193–4, 196
   Woman's Hour (R4) 106, 166
BDSM 76, 110, 169, 245
Beauvoir, Simone de 122
Beech, Cally Jane 190
Bertin Review (2025) 235–7
bestiality 106, 132, 168, 169, 224
Beyond Equality 241
'Big Black Cock' 96
Big Porn–Big Tech collusion 38–43, 47
Big Tech:
   metaverse 200
   non-consensual material 165, 185
   online safety 227, 229, 233–4
   and our algorithmically curated lives 31–4

racial bias 103
turning the tide 241–2
VR and 212, 214
women's speech and rights 20
Black men 41, 91, 92, 95–6
Black performers 97, 101
Black Sexual Economies Collective 100
Black women/girls 91–104
   abuse and 65–6, 87, 182, 187, 193, 221
   Google's racial bias 103
   impacts of racialised 12, 99–100
#BlackLivesMatter 102, 119
Bluesky 27
Boreman, Linda 80
Bose, Adrija 165
Bows, Hannah 169
brain damage 106, 109–11, 120
Brindley, Sandy 167
British Board of Film Classification (BBFC) 9
brown women/girls 37, 66, 94, 102
Burgess, Matt 163, 164

Cameron, David 168–9
Canada 218, 225, 226
'casting couch' genre 162–3
centrefolds, nude 7, 47, 184
Chambers, Chrissy 215–17
chat rooms 42
ChatGPT 221
child sexual abuse:
   anime 94
   children of Pornhub 29–31

315

deepfakes 185
easy access to 8, 35, 59–60
incest 141–61
regulation 28, 224–6
VR and 209–10
See also 'barely legal' porn; incest
Children's Commissioner, UK 46, 57, 172
'the chilling' (UN) 193
choking/strangulation 105–23
   influence of 7, 114–15
   influencers and 39, 42–3
   parallel universes 118–20
   'plastic bag breathplay extreme' 112–14
   regulation 224
   teen example 138
Citron, Danielle Keats 190, 197
civil law reform 215–21
climate change 54, 67
coercion 41, 74, 80, 83, 87, 96, 157, 162, 225
Cole, Samantha 183, 198
Collins, Patricia Hill 92
community forums 37, 61
condom removal 173–4
consequences, VR 209–13
controlling platforms 226–33
copyright, image 34, 191, 215, 217, 218
Coutts, Graham 105–6
Craig, Elaine 48, 49, 157
Crown Prosecution Service 108
cuckolding, interracial 95
'cultural harm' (definition) 63

cultural harms 18, 29, 63–6, 133
'cum shot' 80
'cum tributes' 81, 221
cyber-brothels 204

DaboinkVR 206
dark web 28, 131
Davies, Jess 187, 193–4, 196
de la Peña, Nonny 207
Deep Throat (1970s film) 80
'deepfake porn' 2, 180–99
deepfake sexual abuse 11–12, 20, 64, 94, 163–4, 221, 247
'Deepfakes' 180–1, 183, 187
dehumanisation 4, 93, 97, 99, 114, 244
denial (incest) 145–6, 159, 160–1
desensitisation 9, 131
desire, liberating 22–3
'device-level' age restrictions 230–1
Digital Services Act, EU (2022) 31, 33
'direct effects' debates 61–2
Discord 212
dolls, sex 204
domestic abuse 107, 108, 119
downblousing 20
'doxing' 197
drugging 43, 123, 167, 171, 174–5
Dworkin, Andrea 6, 21, 219
'dysfunctional family' models 144

education, sex 52, 102, 132, 147, 158, 240–1
Eilish, Billie 45

INDEX

ejaculation
  facial 80–1, 243
  photo 221
Emma (on being choked) 116
'empathy machine' (VR) 205, 206–9
End Violence Against Women 168, 220
engagement, participatory 37
erectile dysfunction 63
'erotica' 5–6, 61
Esquire magazine 150
ethical porn creators 34–5
European Commission 31
European Union (EU) 31, 197, 224, 227
exoticism 66, 97
exploitation
  child sexual 210
  as entertainment 86–8, 185–7, 235
  family ties 159
  feminist view 5–6, 21–2
  Mill on 17–18
  minority ethnic groups 98, 100
  profits from 29
exploited-bitches website 168
extreme to mainstream 7–10

Facebook (Meta) 32, 33, 201
facial ejaculation 80–1, 243
Faithfull, Lucy 131, 135
family ties, *see* incest 141–61
'fantasy', beyond 10–12
feminism 21–2, 61–2, 144
feminist critiques 5–7
'feminist' porn 237–40

fetish (definition) 7
fetishes 42, 65–6
fighting back 12–17, 215–42
'fleshlight' 203
Floyd, George 102, 119
'force' porn 1–2, 9, 170–3, 231–2
forgeries, sexual digital 197
Francis, Pope 21
Franks, Mary Ann 197, 248
free porn websites 34–5
freedom and desire, reclaiming sexual 17–19, 243–9
Freud, Sigmund 143

Gadot, Gal 180
Gallop, Cindy 239
Game of Thrones (TV series) 149–50
gay porn 28
Gen Z women 46
gender equality 40, 64, 221, 238
Girls Do Porn 162–4, 217
Glamour magazine 16, 220
Glitch 99
'golden mean', finding the 21–2
Google:
  'barely legal' 129, 136
  'deepfake porn' 2
  executives 32
  facilitating easy access 26–7
  'force porn' 1–2
  'hidden cam' 86
incest 141, 153, 224
non-consensual material 165–6
'nudify' apps 184
online safety 231

racial bias 103
rape porn 1, 169, 170, 178
'sleep porn' 170, 175
grooming 22, 129, 147, 152, 159, 210, 225

haptic technologies (VR) 203
harassment 51–2, 59, 65, 218
Harlow, Jack, 'Lovin on Me' 119
Harrison, Georgia 217
'hatewank' 81
Haugen, Frances 32
health risks 82–3, 119–20
    choking/strangulation 106, 109–12, 122
Hefner, Hugh 100
'hijab' porn 91, 98, 187
'honour killing' 182
human rights–women's rights 19–21
Hunter, Cara 191–2
Hustler magazine 149
hypersexualisation 95, 97, 99, 208

Image-Based Abuse Law campaign 220
'image-based sexual abuse' 83–6, 217–18
'immersive journalism' 207
immigrant women 98
incest 141–61
    advertising 35
    deepfakes and 187
    denial and 160–1
    harm beneath the hype 156–9
    landscape of incest porn 148–55

regulation 224–5
understanding 143–8
use of term 9
See also stepfamily labels
incontinence, female 82
Indian girls/teen 93, 127
Indian women/girls 127, 192
'indie porn' 237–40
Indigenous performers 37
inequality, gendered:
    eroticisation of 77, 123
    harmful porn and 18–19, 56, 65–6, 68
    'orgasm inequalities' 89
    porn silences women 246–7
    religion and 21
Instagram 33, 126, 130, 154, 184, 186
Internet Watch Foundation 135
'interracial' 95, 101
IQs 206
Ireland 225
Isaacs, Kate 192–3

'Japanese' scenarios 85, 93, 94, 127
Japanese women/girls 127
Jodie (deepfake sexual abuse) 186, 189
Johansson, Scarlett 180, 181
Jordan, Jessa 102

Khalifa, Mia 98, 187
King Noire 101
Knight, Tyler 101
Korean scenarios 94
Kristof, Nicholas 29–30

INDEX

Lanier, Jaron 32–3
Latina women/girls 12, 97–8, 103
Laura (on being choked) 117
law enforcement settings 87
lead in paint analogy 66–7
lesbian porn 28
LGBTQ+ individuals 40, 66, 182
LinkedIn 184, 199
Literotica 61
Longhurst, Jane 105–6
Lorde, Audre 4, 91, 93
Lucy Faithfull Foundation 131, 135
lung cancer 53–4
Lust, Erika 113, 239

MacKinnon, Catharine 5–6, 21, 219
#MakeLoveNotPorn 239
'manfluencers' 39, 41, 60, 119, 132
manipulation 25, 38–9, 43–4, 157, 236
   See also AI (artificial intelligence)
'manosphere' 38–42
Mastercard 30, 165, 182
men's health website (project) 136
Meta/metaverse 12, 33, 197, 200–14, 201
#MeToo 242
Microsoft 32–3, 185
Mill, John Stuart 17–18
Millane, Grace 78
minority ethnic groups 12, 65–6, 87, 91–104, 182, 193, 221
   See also individual groups

misogynistic content 12, 23, 40–2, 60, 76, 111, 243–4
Monroe, Marilyn 248
Morgan, Lucy 16
Mort, Helen 188–9, 196
MrDeepFakes 2, 163–4, 185, 195
murder, during sex 78, 119
Musk, Elon 177
Muslim women 91, 98, 187

National Center for Missing and Exploited Children, US 131
National Crime Agency, UK 126
nationality 94
necrophilia 106, 149, 224
negative emotions 32
New York Times 134
New Zealand 150, 156–7, 225
Noble, Safiya 103
non-consent 162–79, 180–2, 217, 248
   types of 11, 53, 83–6, 96, 97, 138, 177
non-fatal strangulation 108, 119
Norfolk, Andrew 22
Northern Ireland 191
#NotYourPorn 29, 192–3, 220
'nudify' apps 35, 181, 184, 185
Nussbaum, Martha 18

obscenity laws 223
Ofcom 138–9, 224, 228, 229, 234
'one-way sex' 174
Online Safety Act, Australia (2021) 33–4

Online Safety Act, UK (2023) 33, 170, 178, 224, 226–8, 231
'Online Safety Commission' 233–4
OnlyFans 28–9, 126, 138, 217, 235
orgasms 46, 89, 204
Owen, Baroness 221

paedophilia 130–2
Pakistan 182
Parker, Sean 33
'participatory porn' 37, 47–52
Patreon 210
patriarchy 3–5, 34–8
  consent and 77–9, 106–7, 121
  creating porn without 237–40
  criminalising 223–6
  cultural harm and 18, 64, 133
  end of 248–9
  incest 141–61
  loathes women 244–6
  manosphere and 42, 90
  'public toilet' example 243–4
  'racist' 4, 91
  young women and 137
PayPal 30
Pelicot, Gisèle 174
penises 7, 96, 113, 117, 138, 147, 203
Penthouse magazine 149
performers/actors, porn 36–7
Photoshop 180, 187
'plastic bag breathplay extreme' 112–14
Playboy 7, 47, 100, 183–4, 248
pleasure, women's sexual 88–90, 99–100

pollution 67
porn industry 124–5, 128–9, 219–20
  advertising 200
  'barely legal' 128
  deepfakes 191
  fighting racism in the 23, 100–2
  'interracial rate' 101
  magazines 16, 56, 149, 150, 220
  more rights, fewer risk 235–7
  transformation of 47
Pornhub:
  advertising 200, 212
  algorithms 37, 113–14
  'barely legal' 124, 125, 127–8
  Blacked channel 95
  categories 35
  children of 29–31
  choking/strangulation 113
  community 61
  deepfakes 193
  'force' 1, 172–3
  Girls Do Porn 162–4
  'hidden cam' 86
  incest 149, 150, 153, 154–5, 158
  Isaacs and 192
  lawsuits against 83–4, 125, 163
  online safety 231
  pollution analogy 67
  pop-up warnings 135, 172, 175–6
  PR offensive 30
  regulation and prevention 134–6, 230
  site visits 25, 26, 35
  'sleep' 174–5
  terms of service 113–14, 154–5

INDEX

titles 9, 75
'transparency report' 155
virtual-reality porn 204–5
pornography (definition) 6
prevention, regulation and 134–6, 137–9
prisoners, male 109
privacy rights 20
'pro-porn' 22–3, 67
probability argument 53–5, 67
'problematic sexual behaviours' 58, 63

queer porn 27–8

racism:
  Big Porn and 65–6
  colour coded 91–104
  deepfakes and 182, 187, 193
  fighting racism in the porn industry 23, 100–2
  impacts of racialised sexual scripts 99–100, 101
  mainstreaming 93–8
  making the unacceptable acceptable 102–4
  online abuse 228
  'racist hatewank' 81
  'racist patriarchy' 4, 91
Rackley, Erika 166, 167, 168, 169, 220
rape 59–60, 62, 64, 80, 133, 157, 165–6, 176–7
'rape-adjacent' projection 95
Rape Crisis Scotland 167–8

rape porn 162–79
  criminalising 19
  ethnic minority groups 98, 99
  Google and 1, 169, 170, 178
  relabelled 9
  scenarios 152
  teenagers 171
  titles 129
  what's (still) out there? 170–6
  when rape finally became 'extreme' 166–9
  where now? 178–9
  X/Twitter 169, 176–9, 246
rape-reality website 168
RapePassion 166–7
Reddit 27, 39, 180, 183, 210, 212
regulation 18–20, 220–6
  choking/strangulation 106, 108
  controlling platforms 226–33
  deepfakes 182, 198
  extreme porn 8, 166–9, 167, 224–5, 229
  Image-Based Abuse Law campaign 220
  incest 156
  'intimate intrusions' 222–3
  non-fatal strangulation 108, 119
  and prevention 134–6, 137–9
  rape laws 176
relabelling content 8–9
reputational sabotage 190–1
responsibility, reattributing 142, 145–6, 158, 159
'revenge porn' 215–16

Revenge Porn Helpline, UK 30, 216, 220
Roblox 201
robots, sex 204, 213
'rough sex' 69–90
  aggression 73–5
  anal sex 81–2
  choking/strangulation 105–23
  consent and patriarchy 77–9
  facial ejaculation 80–1
  spitting 75–7
  young people and 8, 71–3, 78–9, 83, 132
Ryberg, Ingrid 238

sabotage, reputational 190–1
Sade, Marquis de 80
schizophrenia patients 109
'schoolgirl' porn 65, 85, 132, 167, 173, 186–7, 209–10, 234
schools 41, 59, 181–2, 189, 233, 240
  See also teenagers
Scotland 167
scripts, sexual 52–6
  consent and 115, 247
  impacts of racialised 97, 99–100, 101
  incest and 157–9, 161
  participatory porn 47–52
  pornographic websites and 61–2
  teens/young people and 132, 137
search engines 23, 106, 126, 165, 199, 218, 231–3
Second Life 209
self-censorship, by women 12

self-harm networks 33
sex education 52, 102, 132, 147, 158, 240–1
'sex-negative' 3, 15, 77, 111
sex-simulator porn games 35
sex-tech market 203–4
sex workers 17, 28, 81, 191, 207–8, 221
sexism 12, 38–9, 64, 65, 234
sexual abuse:
  deepfake 11–12, 20, 64, 94, 163–4
  incest 148
  See also 'barely legal' porn; child sexual abuse
'sexual digital forgeries' 197
sexual harassment/abuse in 59, 65
'sexual integrity' 223
'sexual scripts' 52–6
  consent and 115, 247
  impacts of racialised 97, 99–100, 101
  incest and 157–9, 161
  participatory porn 47–52
  pornographic websites and 61–2
  teens/young people and 132, 137
sexually transmitted infections (STIs) 83
sibling sexual abuse 141, 147–8, 149, 150, 152–3, 161, 176, 187, 225
silence, porn and 3, 182, 191–3, 246–8
Sjööblom, Lena 184
'slavery-era sexual ideologies' 65–6, 92–3, 96, 103

INDEX

'sleep porn' 14, 48–50, 152–3, 170, 172, 174–6, 231–2
'smart' glasses (Meta) 197–8
smartphones 26, 57
Snapchat 27
social media companies 2–3, 133, 218
social media sites 171–2, 184–5
  access to porn 38, 130, 165
  AI and 227
  deepfakes 182, 190, 195, 196
  incest 154
  largest 27
  'participatory porn' 37
sphincter injury, female 82
spitting 75–7
stalking 197, 218
Stardust, Zahra 36–7, 100, 238
'stealthing' 173–4, 231–2
Steinem, Gloria 6
stepdaughter example 47–52
stepfamily labels:
  incest 148, 152, 155
  regulation 225
  sexual scripts example 48–9
  video tags 127, 246
  virtual realities 200, 212, 234
stepson example 153
Stop It Now website 135
strangulation, *see* choking/strangulation
Stripchat 26, 31
Stylist magazine 56
'suffocation' 105–23
suicide 30, 182

Sunday Times, The 125
survivor experiences 84–5, 157
Sweden 223
Swift, Taylor 185
synonyms, labelling and 1–2, 9

Tate, Andrew 39, 119, 246
'teen' porn 28, 74, 124–40, 151
Teenagers:
  AI-generated nudes 189
  Black men and 95
  body image issues 33
  choking/strangulation 115–16, 117, 244–5
  deepfakes and 181–2
  'the girls in porn like it' 57–60
  incest 157, 158
  online porn content studies 69–70
  rape 133
  rape porn websites 171
  sexual assault/rape 59–60
  sexual harassment 65
  Tiktok and 40
  underage girls 49–50
  views on porn 132
  virtual-reality headsets 201
  X/Twitter 27
teledildonics 203
Telegram 186
Telegraph 139
Thai scenarios 93
Thompson, Rachel, *Rough* 72, 117, 118

TikTok:
  AI and 39
  child sexual abuse material 126
  choking/strangulation 120
  incest 154
  'nudify' apps 184
  spitting 76
'time-stop' porn 175
tobacco analogy 53–4, 66
'tolerance' to porn 8–9
Trump, Donald 41, 227
Twitch 27

Ukrainian genre 87
underage girls 49–50, 94, 127
Undress Ai 185
United Nations (UN) 19, 70, 193
United States (US):
  choking/strangulation 116–17
  deepfakes 184, 189, 197
  online safety 227, 229
  rape porn 172
  regulation 218
upskirting 20, 85

vaginas 129, 151, 153
Vera-Gray, Fiona 167, 174, 195
violence, sexual 69–90
  cultural harms 29, 64
  linking porn to 10–12, 245
  risk factors for 59
  See also individual offences
Virt-a-Mate 212
virtual reality (VR) 12
  arousal and 204–6

definition 202–4
'empathy machine' 206–9
false promise of 213–14
headsets 201
porn 200–14
real consequences 209–13
virtual/robot sex 204, 205
VirtualRealPorn 205
Visa 30, 165, 182
voting preferences 41
voyeurism 85–6

'wake-up' porn 47–52
Walker, Alice, 'Coming Apart' 92–3
Walton, Adele Zeynep 33
white men 66, 91, 95, 100
white performers 36, 94, 100
white women/girls 93, 94–8, 96, 103
Women and Equalities Committee, UK 221
women's rights, human rights are 19–21

X/Twitter:
  'barely legal' 124, 129
  deepfakes 185, 192–3
  extreme violence on 114
  facials in profiles 81
  incest 141, 153, 224
  'patriarchal porn' 3
  'public toilet' 243
  rape porn 169, 176–9, 246
  teenagers 27

INDEX

XHamster 47–52, 136, 173, 231
XNXX 26
XVideos 29–31
   categories 172–4
   'hidden cam' 86
   incest 154
   online safety 231
   race/nationality 94, 96
   rape videos 166
   site visits 26
   titles 7, 136, 138
   voyeurism 85

young men 38–42, 57–60
   Beyond Equality 241
   erectile dysfunction 63
   harmful porn and 46
   rape porn and 179
   'rough sex' 73, 132
   virtual-reality porn 204

young women:
   and aggressive sex 56
   'barely legal' 129, 225–6
   Black and minoritised 65–6
   choking/strangulation 106, 111, 120–2, 232
   coercion into pornography 161–6, 235
   deepfake sexual abuse 182, 194–5
   harmful porn and 45–6
   harassment of 51–2
   real-life sex 60, 132
   'rough sex' 71–3, 78–9, 83
   sexual assaults at university 172
   spitting 75
   unwanted sexual encounters 15
   voting preferences 41
   YouTube 38, 39, 119, 190

Zou, Zhenhao 175